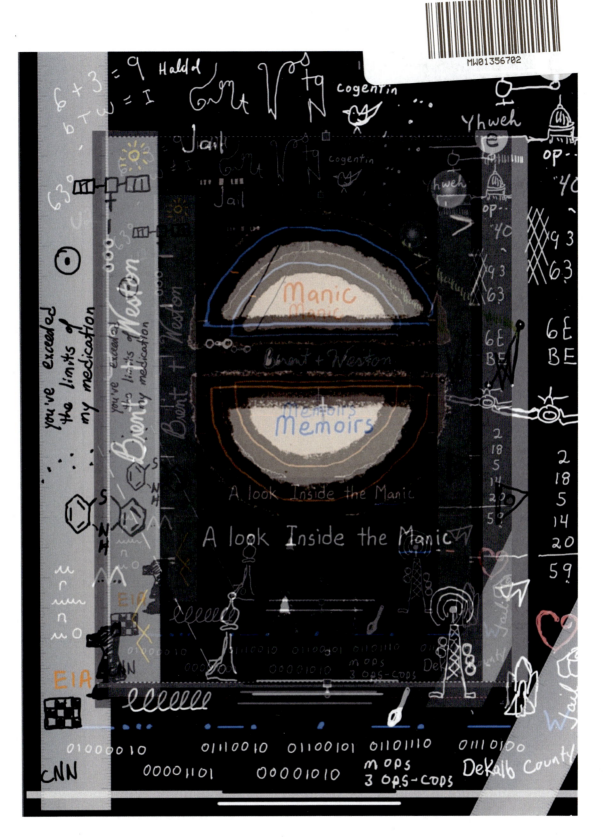

Manic Memoirs

0p-=====].

0p-=====].

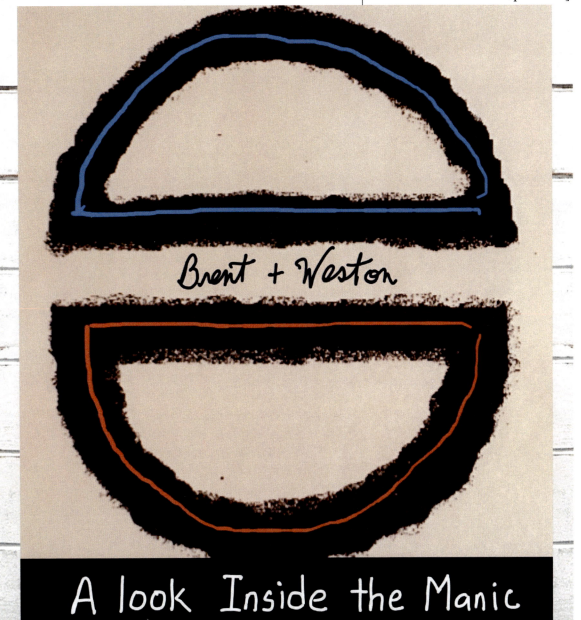

A-rl

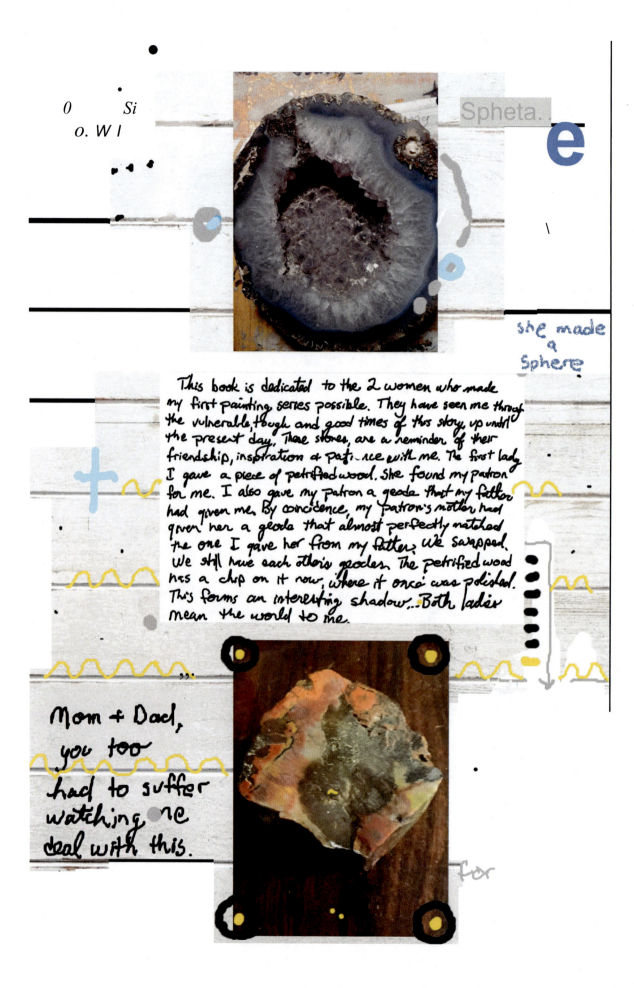

0 Si
o. W 1

Spheta.

e

she made a Sphere

This book is dedicated to the 2 women who made my first painting series possible. They have seen me through the vulnerable, tough and good times of this story, up until the present day. These stones are a reminder of their friendship, inspiration & patience with me. The first lady I gave a piece of petrified wood. She found my patron for me. I also gave my patron a geode that my father had given me. By coincidence, my patron's mother had given her a geode that almost perfectly matched the one I gave her from my father. We swapped. We still have each other's geodes. The petrified wood has a chip on it now, where it once was polished. This forms an interesting shadow... Both ladies mean the world to me.

Mom + Dad, you too had to suffer watching me deal with this.

for

A look Inside The Manic • !''' Art

Story By
Brent T. Weston

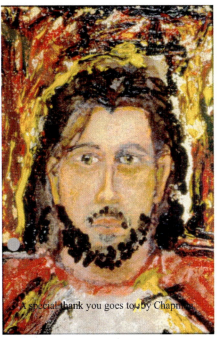

A special thank you goes to Joby Chapman

Based on accurate and inaccurate memories of Brent T. Weston.

REVISED EDITION
June 23, 2019
UNITED STATES COPYRIGHT OFFICE © MARCH 1 6 , 2018

Table

boalt. lt

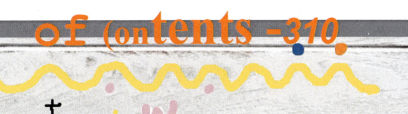

of (ontents -310

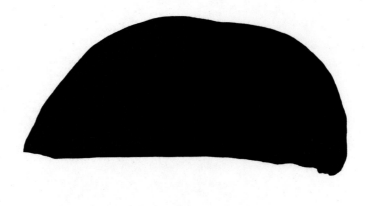

Lowr... :C pu-t "'Y rnof-\0•1»\ec.
milt...s+a,, +N"'o'jk *lt* N?le i

Outlines

A LOOK INSIDE THE MANIC

"Travel Alert" "Manic Memoirs"

The Stages are Set
Techy Teaching
European Year
European Paintings of Foundation
Resting in Restaurants
Pushing Up High on the Rock of Stone Mountain
Manic Intrusion of Marriage Associations

5. Not Sleeping as a Jailbird · 88
6. Flashback to Café Diem · 106
7. Sounds Start and the Orange Glow · 116
8. The Table Turns · 125
9. Bloody Hand at EIA · 129
10. Mental Sounds + Audible Images of People · 137
11. Shadow of Death · 154
12. The Fly, The Zest Wrapper, The Beach, + The Butterflies · 164
13. The Gray Cell of Hell · 184
14. Safe Haven at the State Mental Hospital · 206
15. Chess at EIA · 223
16. Tripping With the People of Airplanes · 230
17. Psychology of the Dark Window · 246
18. Leaving Confinement to Rest in Dad's Lap · 263
19. Hot Coca-Cola In the Tub
20. Baseball at the Private Mental Hospital
21. E and Orangina · 279
22. Surprise at Mailbox · 282
23. Current Artwork

310
24. Final Notes · 294
25. Most Recent Works
26. College Thesis Statement: UTC

Forward

"What's it aawwwllll abbooouuuut?," he asked in his slow, drawn out, broken English with eyes a-buzzing. Awkwardly sipping from his plain, old, white ceramic cup, he never seemed to be looking at us. He was looking somewhere beyond and into the dark. With his quickly vibrating eyes floating in their caverns, he quietly stared, looking right past the sockets of our eyes into the void. Why did I feel compelled to turn and look at the wall behind me? Passing through the windows of my own soul, he could surely see I was a freshman architecture student, scared silly, but absorbing it all in. I felt like a boy and a stranger, carrying an unknown feeling of the sacred amongst the professional teachers who knew their craft of designing buildings and molding young minds.

"What's it all about?" seemed to be the only sentence our new architecture professor at the Georgia Institute of Technology had in his lexicon structure. I kind of felt sorry for him as the green tea leaves, on long stems, were swimming around in the bottom of his mug. He never revealed his life source within the swirling tea. Nor did he ever seem quite happy with our answers to that one question regarding our architecture projects and our lives, "What's it all about?" It was only every now and then, out of nowhere, and usually having nothing to do with us, we got a smile shining to us from the Orient. His lone question was the first at GA Tech that made me think. Rumors were "the one" was a key to it all, but this concept caused my newbie instincts to rail against me. Good and evil are ultimately very real and very separate.

•. "Why are you shaking like a leaf?"

Asks Peter Gabriel through my headphones.

As I ponder why I write and paint, I've been wondering about those words that echo in my ear from nearly thirty-six years ago, "What's it all about?" My stories are simply my art, but on a deeper level, my books are of mental illness. It exposes how my brain does, and does not, work. The books are not typical as compared to most others. They are a whirlwind, and challenge the process of reading itself. There are some words of order and some words of warning.

To start, "A look Inside the Manic, Travel Alert." is chiefly a picture book of my personal paintings. If a picture tells a thousand words, and pictures are generally taken very quickly, then just how many words does a painting represent with all the time that goes into making one? By that measure, this pictorial story is epic. This is the history of a young man who dropped out of the GA Tech Architecture program; a young man who backpacked Europe for two, one-year long trips while feeling the "calling" to be an artist; a young man who returned to GA Tech, and then was fortunate to find a patron to paint a series of restaurants in Atlanta. Travel Alert. is basically images from living the good life, great life... really. I had made early strides to climb the ladder of artistic success, for one in their early twenties. This book simply sets the stage for A look Inside the Manic, Manic Memoirs.

A look Inside the Manic, Manic Memoirs is where my life takes a dramatic turn into mental illness. It slows down into a screenplay format. The original story was written in a screenplay format outlined from a two hour video of myself telling my story. A look Inside the Manic, Manic Memoirs is also infused with art, that I painted, and the art pertains to the story.

As for the words of warning, the books became VERY confusing over a few minutes. I thought I had finished the early writings in entirety. My wife had meticulously checked the spelling and grammar of the screenplay; every comma was in its proper place and every image centered. I venture to say there was not a misspelled word. Then, I ran all my writings through Adobe Acrobat and exported it into Word. I was mortified. It seemed to have changed everything, even the images. However, there were so many inconsistencies as to when the program decided to change the words and images around, that it seemed, in a few places, briefly, like another creative mind was at work.

In Travel Alert., much of my hand written words were reconfigured with Ocular Character Recognition (OCR) Software within Adobe Acrobat. The conversion/ reconfiguration of the OCR will look confusing with jumbled letters and numbers, but are usually derivatives of my handwriting by the computer. The OCR tried to rewrite my handwriting using keys from the keyboard. In some cases, I have put the original text written before the Ocular Character Recognition, under or above the OCR, as to show Adobe's computer derivative interpretation. In other cases, I no longer have the original text, so I had to guess at what I originally had written. In some cases I have actually now turned the OCR into art.

Personally, the more I study the OCR, the more intrigued I get. On the cover page it added the word "Op" from nowhere. Just bizarre! Then, on the title page, I had drawn a yellow circle around the title making a halo over the painted figure. The OCR turned a simple yellow circle into what looks like, to me, a hand with a sword or black light-saber or ruler or a conductor's musical wand, going around the title. HMM? At one point I ask, "Does language have meaning?" and, "Does OCR have meaning?" The computer answered the question with "mos+", under the next painting. On the last typed page of the book, it reconfigured my poem.

The OCR also messed around with the actual typing throughout *Manic Memoirs*. Words have stray letters, spatial gaps, and actual misspellings. It looks like I did not correct my typos. "I"s were made "T"s. Just remember, originally the screenplay was all was correct. In this reworking, I feel the OCR exposed the rhythms of my brain. I rarely think in consistent speeds without some kind of interruption or typographical mistakes. I have given up on 100% editing. The typos and mistakes are possibly closer to certain kinds of truth.

Understandably, for my wife, the OCR ruined all her original editing. The story no longer flows, especially in *Travel Alert*. Matter of fact, the OCR, in most cases, makes her not only indifferent to what she sees, but angry! She no longer understands what either books are about. For me, the OCR opened a can of worms.

The easiest way to read my books is to just read the English where the "language" is accessible. Be patient; you will get the overall gist of the books with the help of the art. Ultimately, there may be no meaning or "mind" in the OCR. I certainly cannot figure out what it all means, but then again, I'm not sure anyone could prove to me that it does not know what it is doing.

Last, I want each page to be a piece of art. If you look at just how diversified and unique God has made this universe, well, it is amazing! My painting gift is, in general terms, two dimensional. As diversified and fragmented as my books may appear, there is a flow intended. It's not just a riddle within a riddle. The stories now show how my mind thinks in recalling events of my past. I now write, design, draw around and within, the perimeters of the OCR. The OCR is my uninvited and unintended guest into the stories, which is irritating and possibly totally irrational. However, as my wife says, I always have a "BUT." In many cases, I think the reader will need to take a seat and consider the meanings bestowed by the OCR, which at times, seems to be moving ahead of us. OCR may be an art form.
I'll make a deal with you. The following short story just happened in my life. It is a microcosm of my approach to seeing mental illness, only it involves someone else's art and not one of my personal paintings. It also involves Morse code instead of OCR. If you find it fascinating, try "reading" my books, as well as absorbing the images of art. It just may be you will find your own "Morse Code."

1

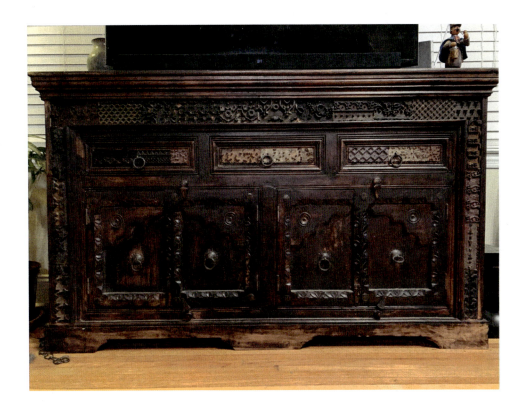

9

―――――

While working at the thrift store that raises money for the local children's foster care, I was routinely carrying in boxes of donated stuff to be separated. It was just another routine day, in a routine week, in a routine month. Bryan, whom I've nicknamed "CB," and Hagan whom I call "Haagen Dazs," both looked at me with excitement. CB said, "You should see what we got in the trailer. We picked it up from under an old house; we pulled it out of a dank basement!" Haagen Dazs chimed in, "It looks like it came off a pirate ship. It's some kind of cabinet or chest or something. It has some really cool ass carvings, dude." If Haagen Dazs says it is cool, it is. He has a pulse on my personal palette when it comes to furniture and clothes. Putting my boxes down, curiosity had me hooked, and my steps were soon following the guys up to the trailer. The eighteen wheel trailer was dark on the inside. CB took the furniture dolly and brought the piece into the store for the manager to price and sell. The chest was being wheeled in vertically instead of its natural horizontal position. At first glance it looked clunky and heavy; the opposite of a light and airy piece of wooden furniture. It looked cumbersome and unloved, covered in cobwebs, but rich with history. CB warned, with a partial laugh, "It could be one of those treasure chests that comes with a curse. Beware and on guard for something bad or funky. I have heard stories and seen movies. You just never know."

Nodding to Haagen Dazs and CB, I smiled an unconvincing smile. Admittedly, though, these eyes had never seen such a piece of furniture. At the thrift store, we do not sell high end furniture because it is only rarely that someone donates an "over the top" nice piece to us. However, there is always the exception, and we do occasionally get an unusual piece that turns our eye. Helping Haagen Dazs carry the piece onto the sales floor, thoughts of this strange piece got sidelined, BUT the longer it sat there, the stranger and more foreign it looked. Checking the decorative panels gave no clue to any of us as to what continent it even came from. The numbers in the drawers were marked in "reverse" order, maybe a clue to being Hebrew or Islamic. The decor just did not add up. Honestly, it did not make sense. Studying iconography for years, in architecture school and two art colleges/universities, did not prepare me for deciphering the markings on this treasure chest. The manager of the thrift store, had no idea either. Recommending to the manager that it needed to be researched before she put a price on it, was advice she surprisingly took. My first inclination was African descent. The archetypal images on the frieze were almost aboriginal. While looking at African furniture on the the phone, ironically an African man came in and offered to buy it on the spot. The manager opted not to sell it until it had been appraised. The African man said he would be back the following week.

That weekend, I got focused on the piece; tunnel vision. Curiosity was overwhelming me. The wooden box was a puzzle. Combing the internet for days looking up every lead possible, left me frazzled. Haagen Dazs spent time on the computer, at his house over the weekend trying to help me in the search. Nothing. Haagen Dazs's mom was also recruited because of her expertise, and come Monday morning, we were all disappointed with our lack of knowledge.

Knowing how unusual the piece was, $300 sounded like a fair price to offer my boss. She, too, thought it fair. One friend offered me advice, "Don't spend more than $150 on it." I had no idea how much it was worth, but wanted to buy it for my home, just for a TV stand. It was a true mystery. I bought it Monday morning for $300 before knowing an actual appraisal. Staring at the overpriced financial purchase I may have just made, I was still happy with the buying of uniqueness. It seemed one of kind, sort of like how I see myself, even though I knew better.

¥

A LOOK INSIDE THE MANIC

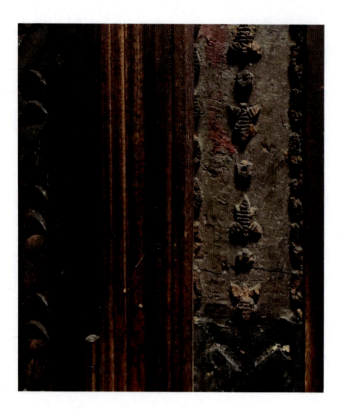

A LOOK INSIDE THE MANIC

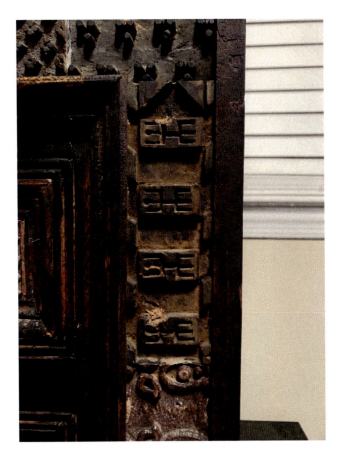

Taking many pictures of the piece from all angles was the first step into my serious research. Step two was to take measurements. Step three was to pay twenty dollars to an online appraiser using my IPhone. The company was chosen because of its reputation with appraisers from well known auction houses. They wrote back that it was a manufactured chest/credenza, more decorative than collectible, maybe teak wood, probably from Zanzibar, value probably $200-$300. They admitted they did not know for sure.

The TV looked great sitting on a clunker of a mystery, and for a week or so the treasure chest eluded my mind. BUT, mental illness gets me focused on one thing or idea, and it is difficult to think about anything else; it is compulsive. In time, it became apparent that many of the archetypal, decorative inlays across the frieze had been removed and/or changed. There was a little residue of recent glue in the cracks. Someone had meticulously done the work.

One night, the glow from lights above the dining room table were illuminating the chest from a distance. Music was pumping rhythmically through my surround sound. Maybe the music was Loreena McKennitt followed by Snow Patrol and Peter Gabriel. Sitting at the table, staring at the dark wood, thoughts of patterns in the patinas intruded into my mind. From where such creative thoughts come from, may just live in the domain of God. It is for sure the patinas had obviously been worked on at great length. It appeared to me that there was something freeing in the removing of the patinas, revealing the underneath. The shapes could breathe. From afar, a Morse Code pattern emerged in my mind. It was going across the front of the piece. The code was where the patina had been removed. Most of my friends do not see it. I have circled what I saw.

Admittedly, it is a weird thing to see. No doubt that conformation bias was also involved. Finding meaning in this piece was paramount and turning into a quest. I had just spent a hunk of change on this box. Rather, my Pops gave me some of the money to buy the credenza. Why a craftsman would spend so much time redoing the inlays kept me baffled. Curiosity and

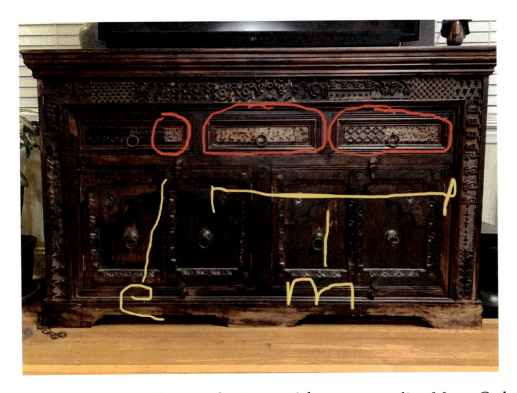

instinct led me to punch E-M, the letters of the corresponding Morse Code on the piece, into Safari on my phone. Immediately, Safari did not pull up a list page of possible sites with definitions and such, but sent me to HTML code. The computer code that just popped up on my screen was later learned to be from the appraisal company. The second word in the HTML was "greeting." Below is the start of two pages of code.

```
{
  "meta": {
    "greeting": "Welcome to Customer.io's edge event collection service. Enjoy your stay."
  },
  "request_endpoints": [
    {
      "GET /unsubscribe": {

...
```

This is freaky to find on your phone after just punching in two letters seen on a piece of furniture; two letters from visual Morse Code. The two letters should have sent me anywhere but back to the website I had used, let alone into their code. To my knowledge, no other two letter combination gets the same reaction on my phone. Obviously, I did not even begin to test all possible two letter combinations.

With questions in hand, immediately my best computer programming friend was given an urgent call. He happens to live in Atlanta, hours away from where I now live. Explaining the situation, asking him why Safari would send me back into computer code from an unknown source and with a "greeting," caused me to go speechless and breathless. He quickly calmed me down and reassured me that it was just "cookies" or something, but he did not know for sure. He admitted it was a little weird. Rambling on about how unusual this piece was and that I could find nothing like it on the web, he interrupted me and told me to just send him a picture of the credenza. He also said he could not talk long because he was currently at his boss's house and he had to go.

Not long after, I got a call back from my friend but now in a serious tone rarely heard from him. He said he had explained my dilemma to his boss, a computer person as well, who may have been even more versed in computer language than my friend. The boss wanted to see the picture of the piece of furniture kind of laughing at the situation. My friend obliged, showing him the picture I had originally sent. The boss then told my friend, "Come upstairs with me." Upstairs was this!

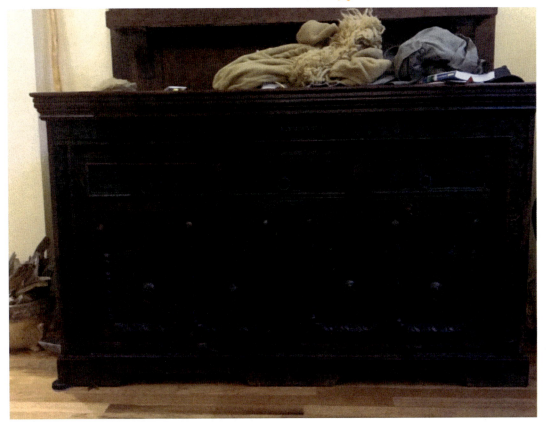

Aslan stone alter

In essence, this is the same manufactured style piece, but the patinas have not been removed from the decorative inlays. His are all blackish. For now, the story ends there, except that my wife's research, along with other friends, has revealed that what was once was thought to be HTML code is actually JSON computer language.

At this point, not putting on any more meaning on the message is paramount so not to lose or loose my senses. It is just just weird and highly unusual, but there are times I still wonder what the JSON is saying. Believing there is a message in the JSON is natural for me, though computer code knowledge is foreign to me. Right now, I am just stupefied with the "greeting."

Part of my mental illness is bestowing personal meaning concerning the physical, conceptual, or spiritual when my paradigm may or may not be correct. Numbers, letters, colors, sounds, vibrations, words, textures, habits of people, anything or anybody can be part of a pattern. My computer friend once said, "It is easier to know patterns than truth." These words haunt me!

One thing I know, patterns, and pattern anomalies, in particular, have been often a "trigger" for my mental illness. It is not easy for me to ascertain when patterns or their anomalies, in an objective world, are made with intention and specifically address me even if only subconsciously. This affects my everyday life; my wife and friends can testify. It is the small questions such as, "Why was the peanut butter left alone by itself on the counter overnight with its label facing out directly at me?" When the visual angles are prominent and relatable, the brand label then becomes a screaming billboard. Then, there is a gap between the thought, "Was the peanut butter accidentally left on the counter?" versus the assumption of a form of possible veridical, person to person, communication. If the angles relate, and I discern a form of communication, I am then looking for meaning and what depth it came from. For example, is it just the designer/maker of the label speaking to me, or is the person who left the peanut butter on the counter communicating a message to me? If I do believe someone left me a message on purpose by the positioning of an object, I see it as poetry with meaning. I face these decisions every day, but at different frequencies and levels of consciousness. The frequency of these types of thoughts, at times, has intervened, become compulsive, and affected my choices, decisions, and actions. This is especially so when synchronistic events introduce themselves as thought players on the mind's stage.

When current synchronistic events connect with the residue of past, layered synchronistic memories, an internal language begins. From the chasms of thought, there is birth and form. It is also here, where over the recent years, I have learned patience to slow the thoughts down and bring them before God. I used to see synchronicity as a real sign from God to be quickly, and urgently, followed. I try to be more careful now. How this all first crazily played out in 1994, the year of my first real manic break, is revealed in *Manic Memoirs*, and written in much more simple words. Thank God, yesterday is gone. Today, it is just easier to say: Maybe, I'll make a peanut butter and jelly sandwich.

Surprisingly, precisely because there was not a pattern in Adobe's reconfiguration of my first two books, there was a significant "trigger." The oddity with no pattern, first appeared as a total mess, then suspiciously serendipitous, and then as art, creative and disruptive. This provokes an important question for me in my first two books: "How far do I explore Adobe's conversion that affected my writing and page templates?"

I do have questions for Adobe. The first question I have is concerning the OCR. Why did it add some cryptic code-like characters into my script from pages that had nothing? In its additions, OCR went beyond just translating what I had written. However, the second question I have for Adobe is why did the program recreate my page boundary frames? Since *Manic Memoirs* involves being incarcerated, I wanted each page to look like, and feel, the repetition of white cells within a jail. An architectural line drawing of a single box cell around the words and paintings was intentional on my part. Adobe changed and altered the look of the architectural drawing for almost every page. The changes appear uniquely catered to the individual page and, thus, now more compositionally mysterious. This is more than my expertise could or would ever do. It feels like someone "hacked" into my cell template and made them more uniquely designed. How this was done, I have no idea! It just seems the sum of these changes is intentional.

Is this intuition about my story being "hacked" for the compositional betterment, mental illness? I do have to admit Adobe's changes could be all random chance playing out its effect in a physical universe at the time I experience it. BUT, this hacking question resembles a deeper question that resonates and is intertwined with my mental illness. Is there an unknown author helping create my first two books? I will not and can not prove to anyone that another author has helped. BUT, I know my a priori towards life directly affects how I believe what happened on the computer.

My a priori and world-view allow for this co-creator mentality. I am often looking for that extra meaning, the underlying current, a foundation for the belief, what is underneath, and am using my epistemological lenses to decipher what is within and around me. After all my years, here are a few bedrock ideas that have generated coordinates for my life. I am an artist. I can create. I can also look at a painting or book, hear a song, see a dance, or experience life within nature, and know there is an Author/ Maker to it all. There is a live being outside of myself who can make art for me to ponder. On a grander scale, the universe, time, and humankind itself are all art. It's the old story that asks whether a clock can form itself. I understand the clock's origin is debatable. The clock also involves mechanical engineering instead of biological engineering. BUT, the a priori for me, and I believe for you, should be that the universe and most of what we know, including life itself, is created with levels of intent. Simply put, the universe and life were made with meaning. Questions of the origin of DNA, the known universe, the concept of infinite bookends, the Golden Mean, animate and inanimate symmetry, and life beginning from seed, are too great not to attribute to a Prime Maker. For me, there is an ultimate, eternal Artist, and that Artist is God. In all respects, I fall short and pale in comparison to the Person who made the universe.

At times, an overwhelming separation from knowing the ultimate Creator intimately has been very real, as *Manic Memoirs* will attest. I feel a similarity of separation with those who changed my books with possible intent. I do ultimately believe separation from God is a result of my brokenness, my ignorance, my selfishness, my choosing, my running away, my hiding, and my pride. Regarding my books, I am lacking the knowledge to make an honest assessment of the possible ghostwriter/artist. With God, there is a spark, a nudge, to continually bow to the greatest Person who ever was, is, and will always be; The "I Am That I Am." This bowing is done in humility, respect, and honor, all for a relationship with my maker. God has revealed to me Jesus is love, Jesus is the ultimate Redeemer, and that we are called to love one another as He has loved us. Regarding the possible hidden ghost/writer, with great fullness of heart, I thank that person(s) for making my book infinitely more compositionally beautiful and unique. I could have accepted what Adobe changed was purely accidental and unintentional, BUT now I want to believe, and I choose to believe, Adobe OCR had a purposeful creative influence on my books. My books are the wedding of art and new technology, and not all done completely by me.

Adobe unlocked the visually bland similarity that runs through many book pages. I am generally overwhelmed by many words sitting on a page; page after page, book after book, library after library. Personal concentration for reading long periods has left me, possibly due to my use of cell phones and other electronic devices. Looking back through my history, though, I have never been much of a reader. I am, after all, a painter by "calling" and by trade. It may be argued what Adobe recreated, rectified a need in my soul. My books had become static and stale; now, they are dynamic! Mystery has returned. Down deep, I was looking for help, some kind of artful breathing space within my story. I felt the story was bound too repetitively in its visual structure. Adobe fixed this for me without me asking. By repercussion, my books are now more kin to magazines and periodicals, and maybe closer to "click bate." This is both good and bad.

Finally, *Travel Alert* and *Manic Memoirs* challenge my own belief in the degrees that technology and art can cohabitate. I find myself considering the various angles and vectors of thought, all the while, trying to maintain a relationship with the Personal God. This combination has produced a lifetime of questions. Much, within these books, will be indecipherable. Maybe that chaos is fertile ground for creativity to flow. Some undefined material may still be good. Is the book a puzzle? I do believe so, and it is a book to learn from. For certain, as you will see, I have written these stories and imbedded these images with the help of a computer on various levels. This computer and its programs were created by people. On one platform, my books are stories and paintings of travel, mental illness, and faith, all while dealing with OCR from the way I have perceived it. Later in *Manic Memoirs*, the platform within the story itself shifts to questions of Artificial Intelligence and the mind. To what level the computer has contributed, or what other minds/Spirit(s) are at play, I leave up to you!

A. Brent

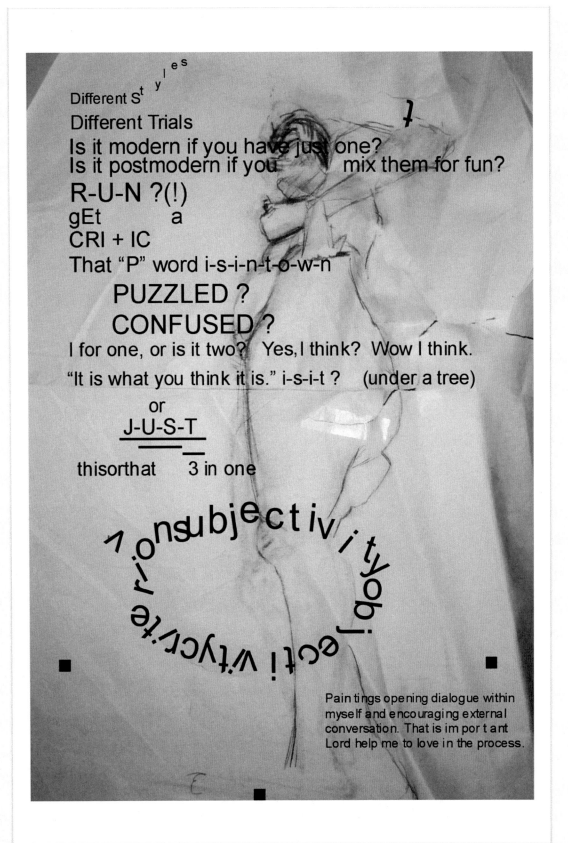

What attributes of PostModernism can fit with Christian worldview?

INT. BRENT'S BEDROOM (BRENT'S RENTED HOUSE)   **NIGHT**

A young man bends over and takes off his sandals, then sits on the floor with eyes abuzz. [Focus on sandals in corner.] They are river "Jesus" sandals made of leather and thick brown shoe laces. The man is in his mid-twenties, slim, and his shoulder-length, dark hair is pulled back in a loose ponytail. His hair is starting to dread. Fingers are wrapped around a pencil. His hand flies across the page of a black bound journal. Low, yellow, brownish light surrounds the bed as the darknesses of night descend across the windows. At one point, as Brent is writing, the shadow of his hand looks like a rabbit smoking a cigarette.

The floor is covered with scenes of interiors from Atlanta's historical restaurants, mixed with some attempts at abstracts. There is a large jar of Benzoate of Soda on a small end table. Contained pigments are placed across the room. A respirator with filters lies on the floor next to a painting of a Waffle House.

                    BRENT WESTON (VO)
There is a time in every searching artist when they begin to wonder just what the hell they are looking at. In '94, I had recently returned from two one year trips backpacking Europe. Milking cows and making cheese high in the Swiss Alps for a summer, was one of many of my crazy adventures. More importantly, at L'Abri, I had built my first easel out of a stolen, old opera singer's walking stick, a kid's spear, some cut wood, an old coffee pot and my bandana. I learned to paint on the streets of Europe and traveled by selling artwork. Now that I had returned home to the South, I had my first art patron. The long hours of painting stage like scenes of interior, historic eating establishments began to wear on me, and I started questioning where to walk on 2

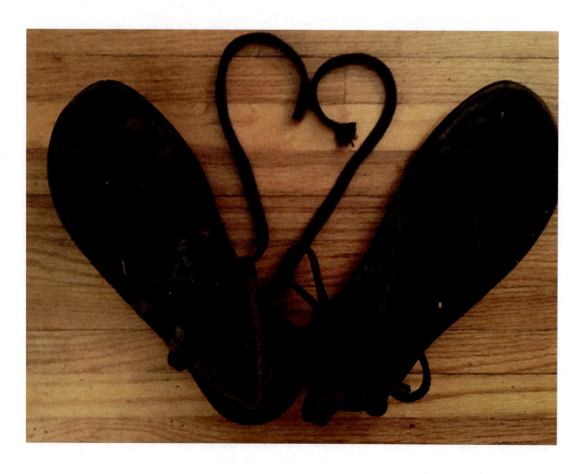

Ga. Tech '93

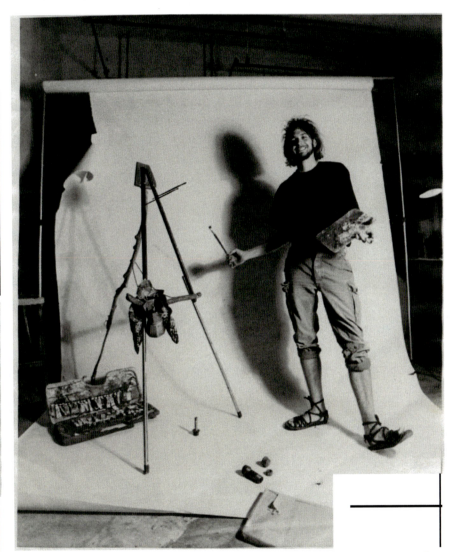

Rambling Wreck from GaTech, let us go for a plod

Shadows were painting on easel.

WGI.scul   c,,ws.,,d
           cJr0&1111inj
for   d\1- 0" +"'e,   f4fff
a

On my first trip to Europe

Parting with the friend I had been traveling with for three months was sad, but necessary. We had traveled from the Isle of Skye in Northern Scotland, through England, Wales, Ireland, France, Spain, Portugal, Spain, Morocco, Spain, France, Italy, Greece, Turkey, Greece, Italy, Austria, Germany to Switzerland. In the pouring rain under some scaffolding in Zurich, we parted ways. It had been an extravagant expenditure; a once in a life time trip, full of adventure and good fun. It was also exhausting and trying.

My remaining travel money was spent to go see a region of Switzerland written about in the book *Let's Go Europe*. "Alone time," or, "down-time" was needed before going home. Hiking down near the Jungfrau was the most breathtaking hike I had ever taken. Stopping to get some ice cream on the hike was a necessary break. Curiously, I asked the lady if she knew of a local cheese farmer that could use help for the summer milking cows. She said to come back in three days. After three days, I was driven up the mountain to a family with five kids, and they did not speak English. This American, of course, did not speak Swiss-German. That started the happiest summer of my life.

Living on Grosse Sheidegg

Within the first 10 minutes of me learning to milk cows, I put my monopoled milk stod through a hole in the floor. I braced my descent with hand in (to) warm cow dung.

"Show me a garden bursting into life"

"This could be the very minute"

I was stuck & had to offer the professional farmer my hand of ✽✝□✦ to be pulled up, out of floor

wr *efipe ie*

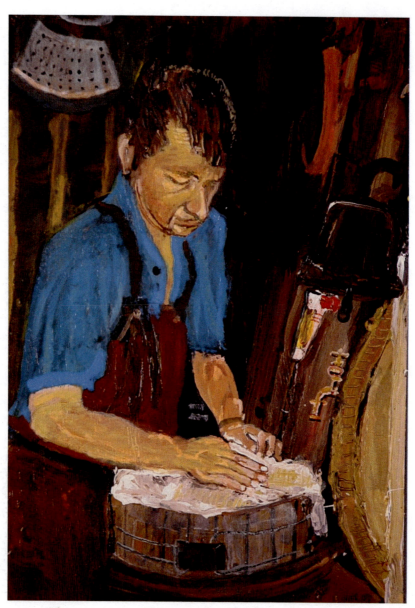

20 Thank you Hans & family for the summer of a life time.

nQdI

Making Real Swiss Cheese

Outside The flies were infinite

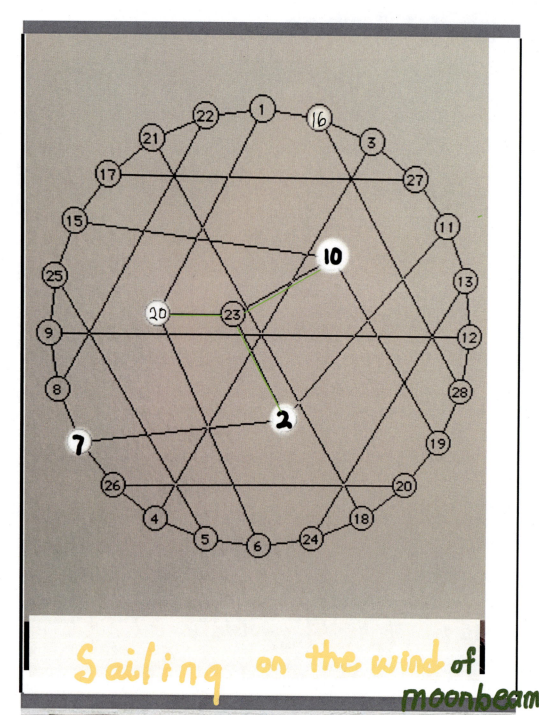

Sailing on the wind of moonbeams

~~Flying~~ on the Radar

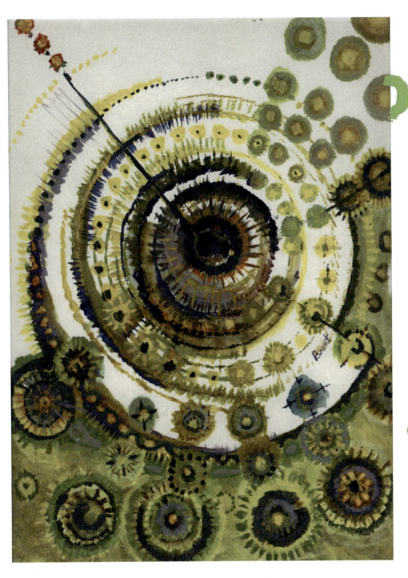

"Swiss first Kiss"

H,"Jt; Ir

Swisher Jumpshot   Swiss Hiking

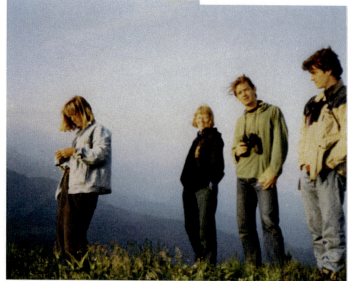

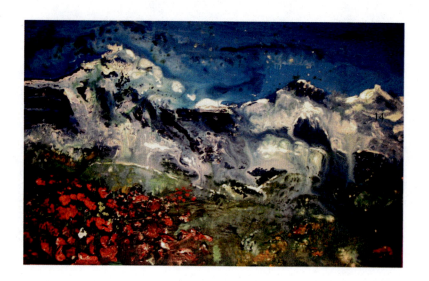

• Photo - near L'Abri in Huemoz, Switzerland

Eiger Monk/Jungfrau ᴍᴍ

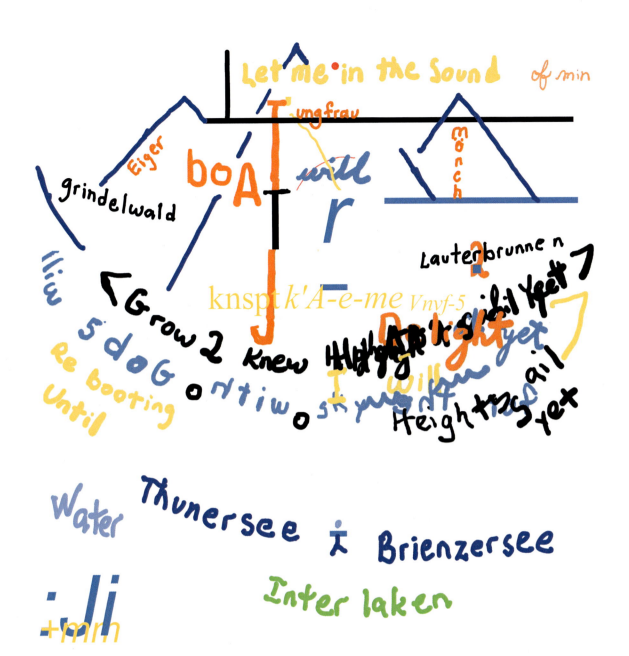

Heigh T S ail yet

li:oo.. 7:oo ttm   a
weak,.

Lvcky
ot   pers6'hd

S+-rea.t &r1M

=

.t

βho-1-os.

Always wanted to go sailing in Interlaken Switzerland

?
/

Dam

Knoc_,k 1\nod

l(noc. "IIId

(DAOI) Lo""-. *Loc.h*

S ai l

(Loe.Ii). away · ll   n

O

On.   Sailing takes me away to where I'm always yearning

to   be.

The CANVAS can do miracles.

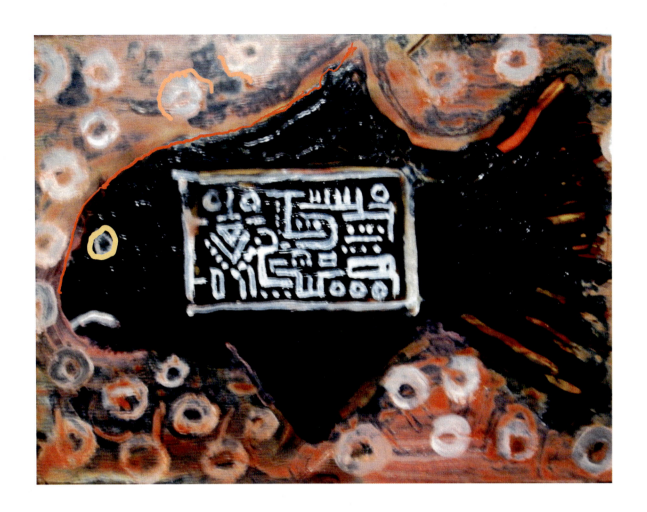

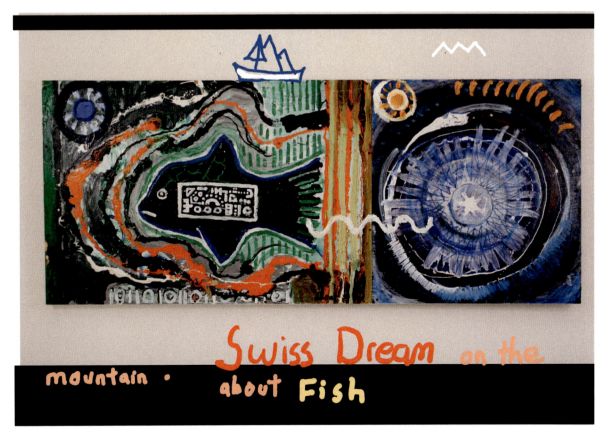

Swiss Dream on the mountain about Fish

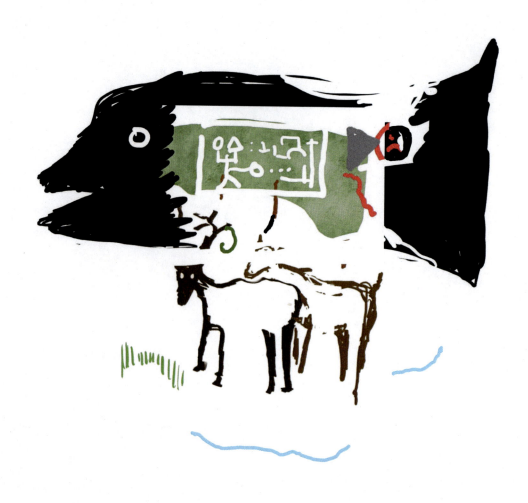

Fish + Steinbach + Berg Widder

ve,
frogs and toads

d{'Jj-S4 *fro3* S

c   *+vads*

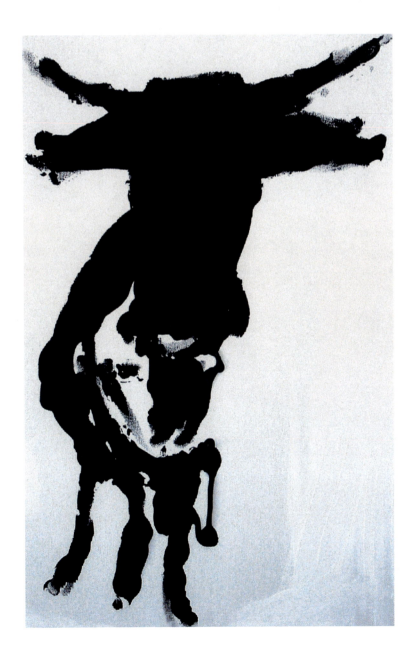

e:

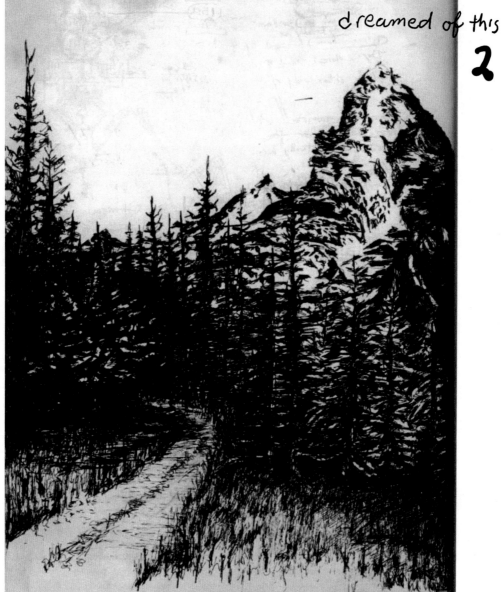

dreamed of this
2

From my journal - Near Grosse Sheidegg · Grindelwald CH

milk farming & cheese
ma stretching

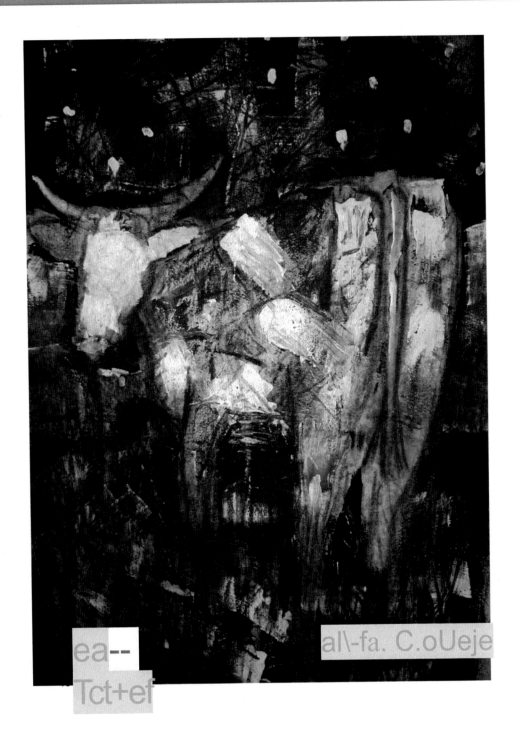

ea-- al\-fa. C.oUeje
Tct+ef

Painted

in Art school
of Art

**V .., go-I' o,
etGCl. drqwlnj**

2 times daily (or more)
Mistschaufel

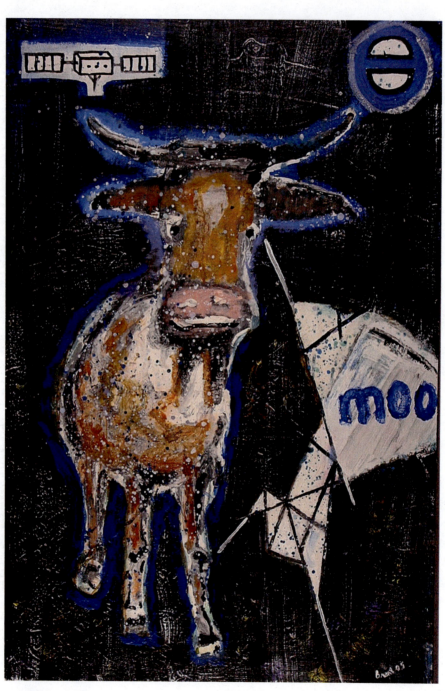

m·. e

Near Unterer Grindelwaldgletscher

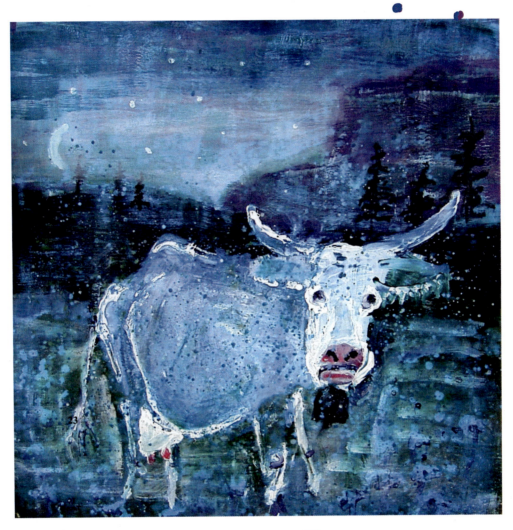

Blve. moonJ

Beyond the Dream

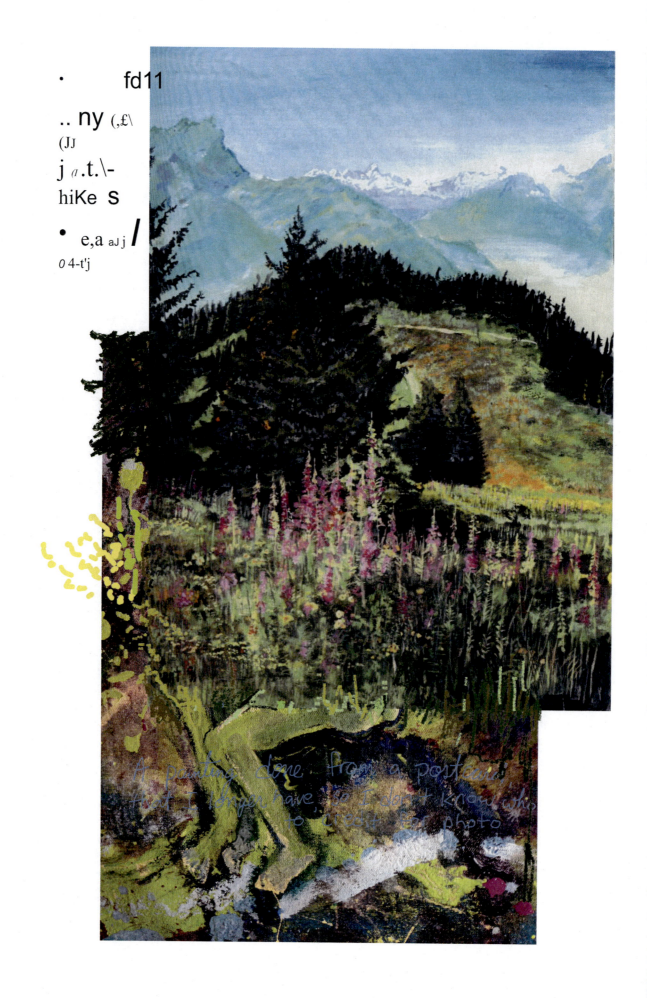

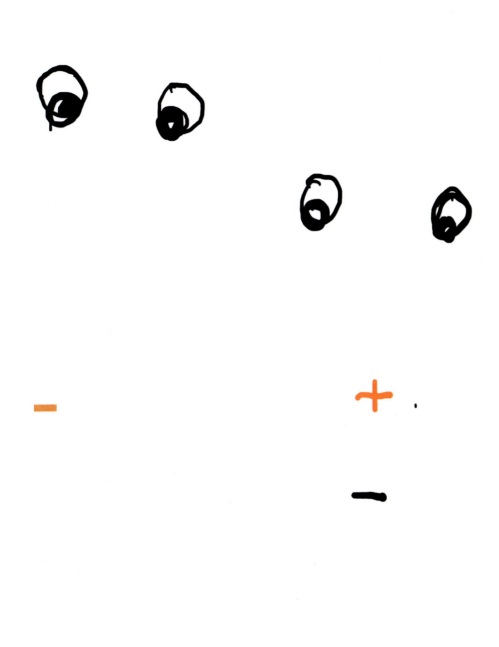

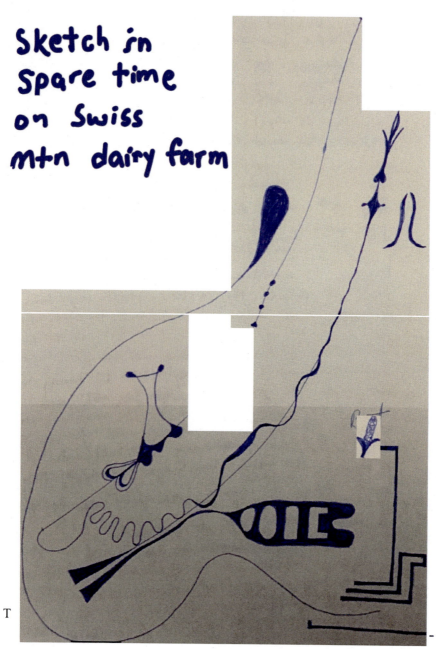

Sketch in spare time on Swiss mtn dairy farm

a. r&,1Y1   u"   LUrH-t M+ure

ll   c-   fl"O   ((,n,   cheese_   wor k

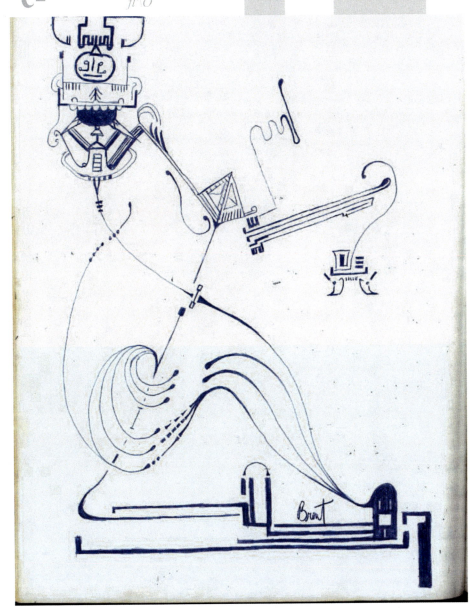

I never shovele d so much shit, but never had so much fun.

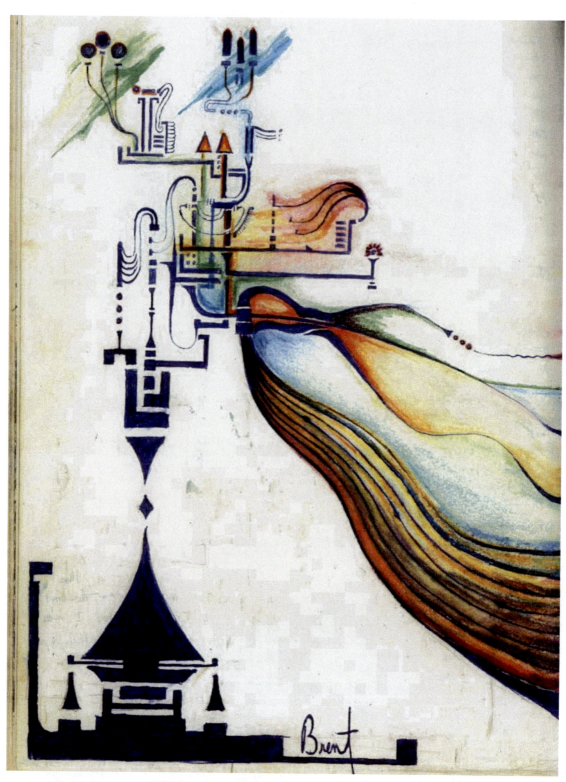

After milking cows — worked on Jungfraujoch — had a Swiss Bank Account — Returned back to USA for a little while

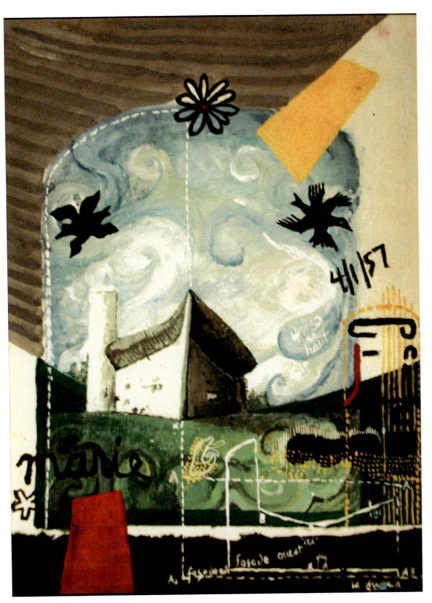

then I WENT BACK...

The second trip to Europe, L'Abri was the place for me to go to study Christianity and the arts. After three months, it proved fruitful. I built an easel, and hitch-hiked to Monzambano, Italy. Renting a house in the Italian countryside off of SP74, my painting started with intention of being an artist for life. The next set of images are mostly from the following 9 months of traveling across Italy, back up to the Swiss town where I had milked cows, and then on to France. This time, paintings were to be my journal.

2. European Paintings of Foundation

The are Fallow Taught Artist my traveling Europe

"early stages"

5e/f

After marrying into being a painter, while at L'Abri, I hitched to Italy + rented a house in a small town to start smearing pigments

Plato's Cow Cave

became the past   StJL.
G-   "4,,,. ,r1ere,
oiqt   Go1o11ht.ll.

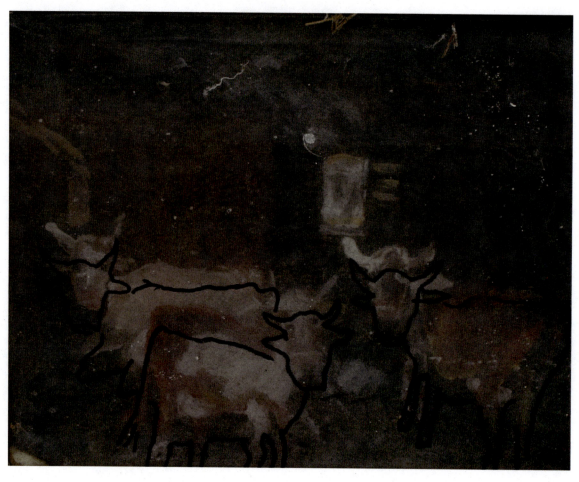

#«h

f)Ott\t.   -9VMf.s+II/-P.
I was now at L'Abri!

.PaUrt w CJ

Dc::J

\+

Co-PfJee Pot'''

I went to the local carpenter shop in Villar above Huemoz, Ch. They wanted over 200 Sf to build an easel. I said I'd try and build one myself. He gave me some wood. Thank You!

CH = Switzerland   Sf = Swiss francs

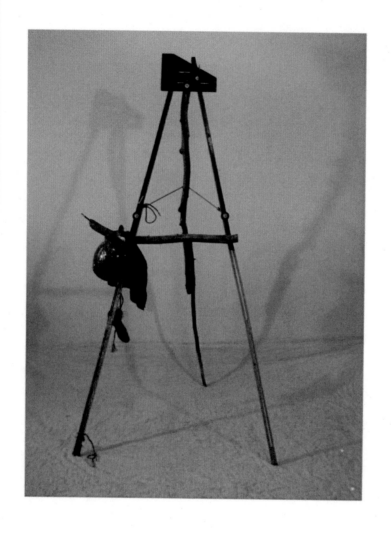

Built in '91. I still [ocasions?]
today

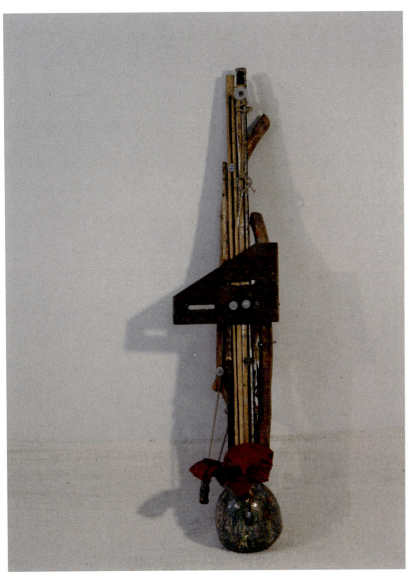

Easel Travel Mode

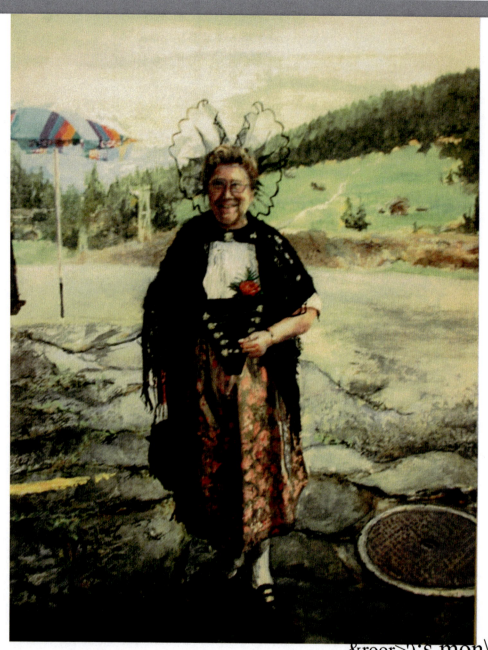

A+ the J\ov.se, in fY\.ol\ bGnt>, *this was* groom's mom
first painting I did. my ow. rJl:P,r>Jsly m
"t\l?. ,:4,,my', o-tO' .. 8e-nv'f-i'hi l l) Crf.,My
first painting in Monzambano. It was from a photo of A Swiss
Groom's Mom at her son's wedding. Later... given as a wedding

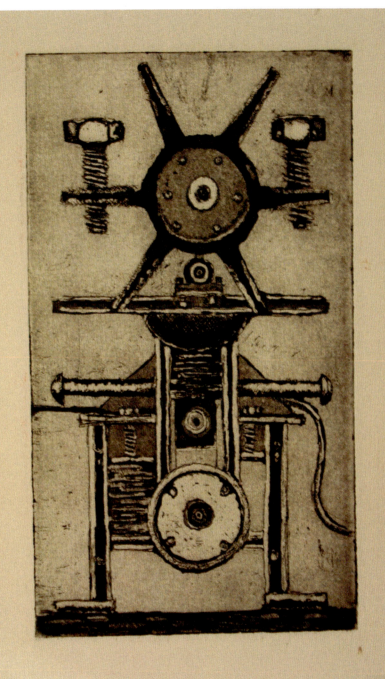

Not bad for a first etching
"got to stand up straight"

36

TY.
U2
SB

present.

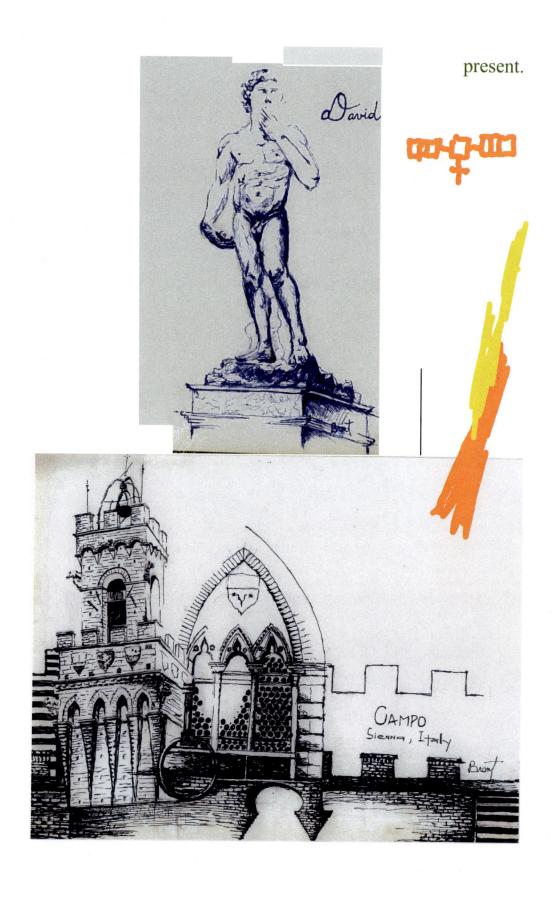

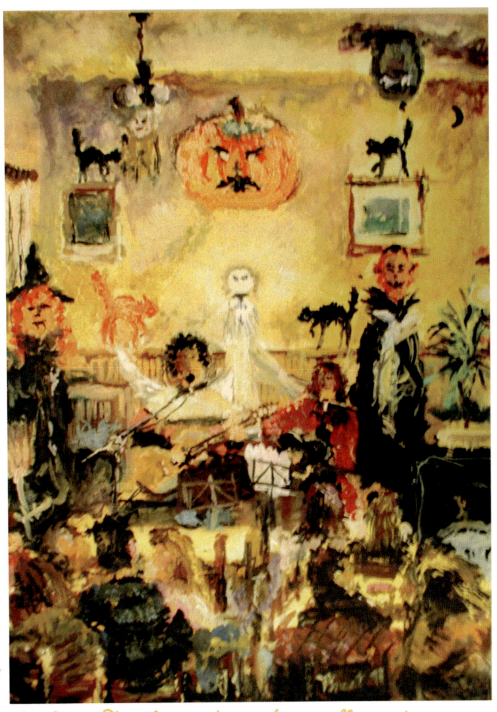

· My first Plein Air painting... done in Monzambano. ·

The local Italians challenged me to get out of the studio in the house I was renting and paint "live"

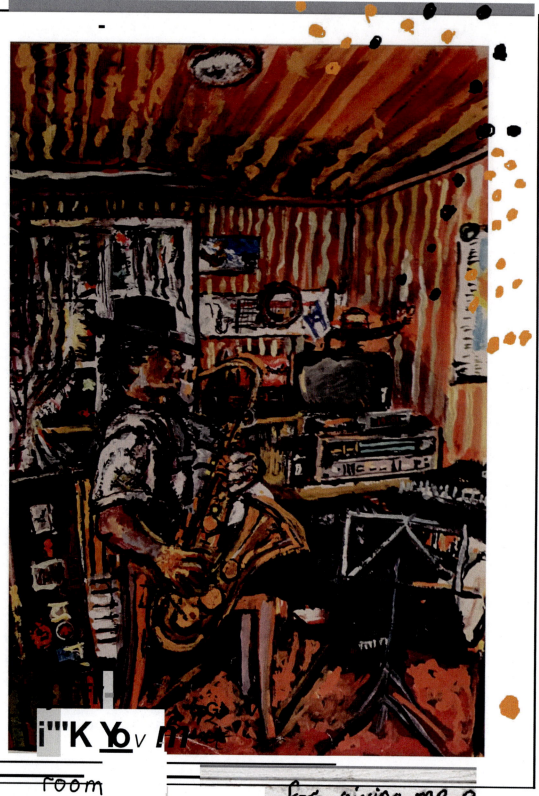

i'"K Yo v m
room   for giving me a
chance to hear Peter Gabriel's "Passion"

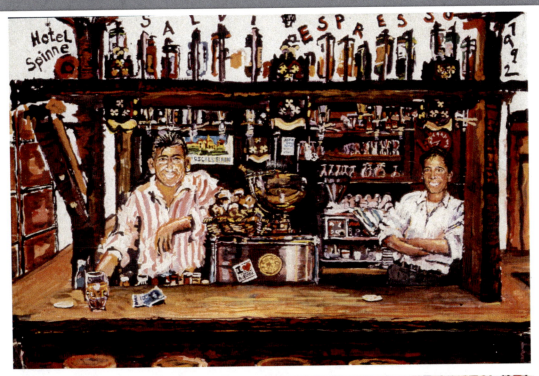
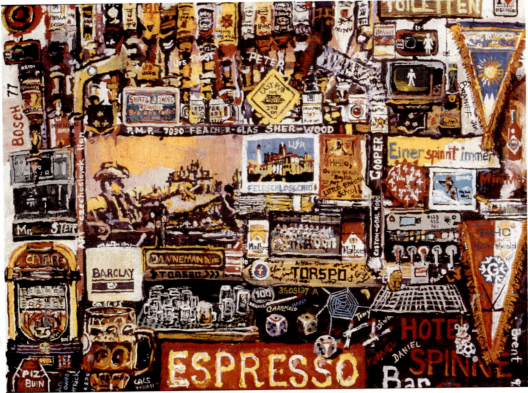

I   f(. A
lady from
UK
Royalty
spilled her
wine on
Espresso
painting,
almost
ruining it
by trying
to daub it
u

a

s,."61.

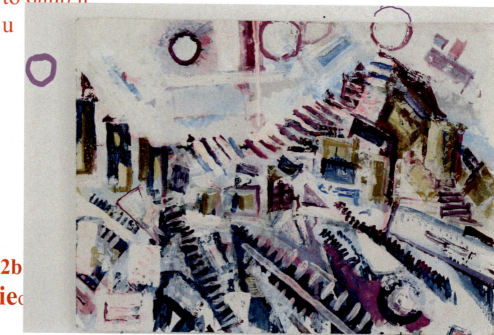

. A11 **i'A2b**
hv ""'tied

Facing Obstacl

Art

Royalty
A member of the Royal Family spilled her wine on the Espresso Bar Painting. She tried to dab it up and almost ruined the whole painting. had to let it dry until paint seeped through. Help

Travels
Sell copies to help pay for my travels.

Eiger
Painted the Eiger in a snowstorm while on the Bunny Slopes. My paints started to freeze.

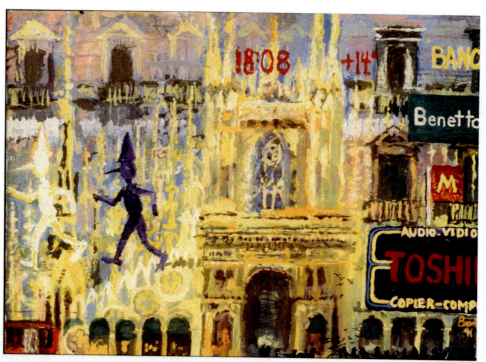

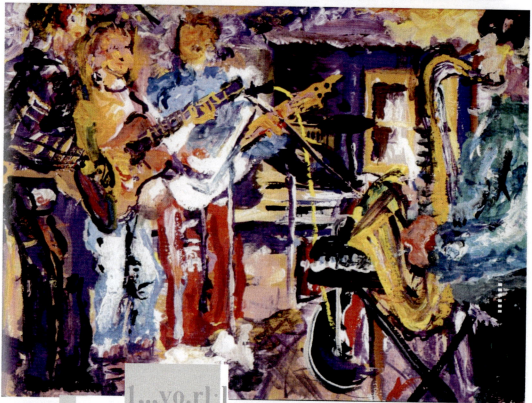

ever o ld, pQin

have been my first
I still haven't found
what I'm looking for

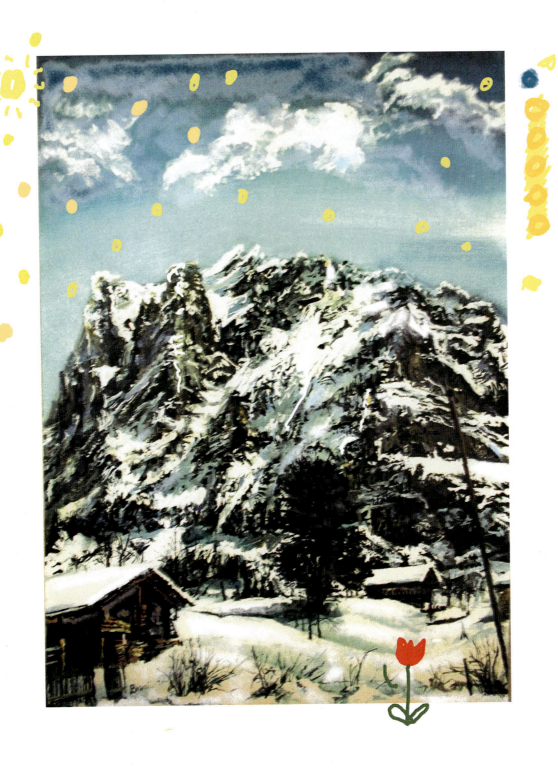

d on e. \ive,ll tor +he *tuf:* of ;t.

in honor of Meni

When thinking of you, I remember the first Red Tulip showing off after a long winter snow

Sorry for temporarily driving off with your car. It was not a funny joke.

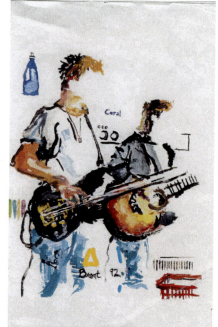

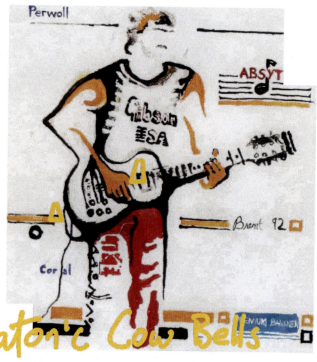

Platonic Cow Bells

I would practice painting while band members practiced. CH

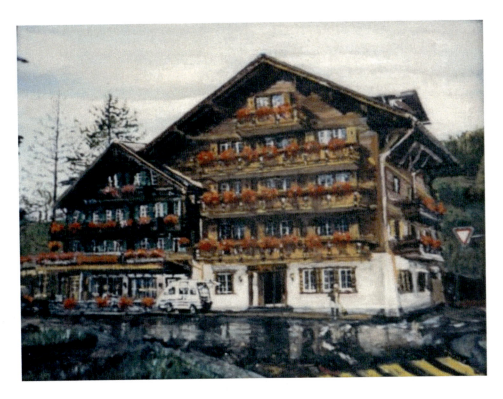

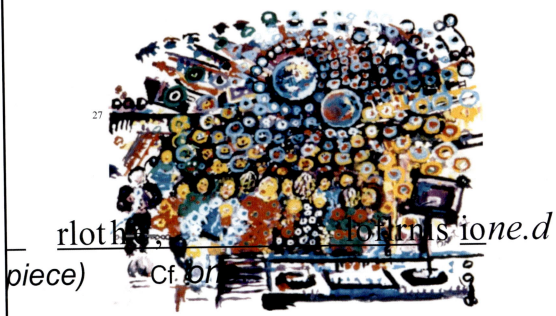

27

rloth-e, lofirnis io*ne.d*
piece) cf *br*

Because of you, I saw rocks as art. Later when I had a patron, I gave her a geode that my father had given me. The next time I saw her, she showed me an identical one in size, color, shape... She put them together to form a sphere. My hair went static.

Her mother had given her the identical matching geode

33 Thank You Bruno! You taught passion of art & life!

and the coffee & pasta Bellissima

Bruno You Rock!

You could make art out of anything

my wife recently did this painting of my patron's Geode. Pottery plate.

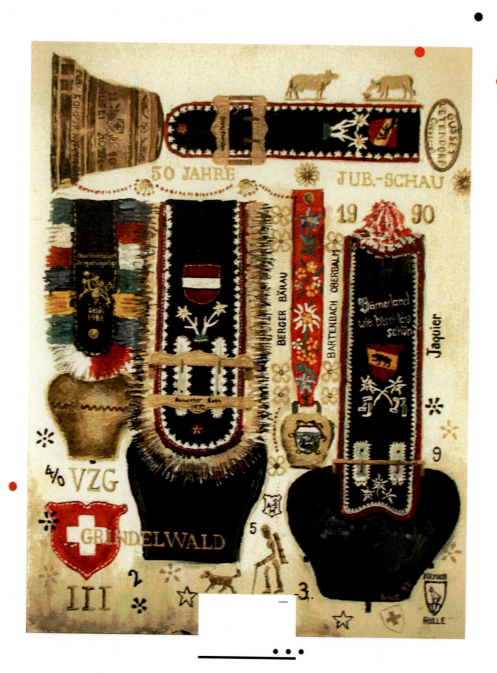

34. "Gotta have more cowbell!" SNL

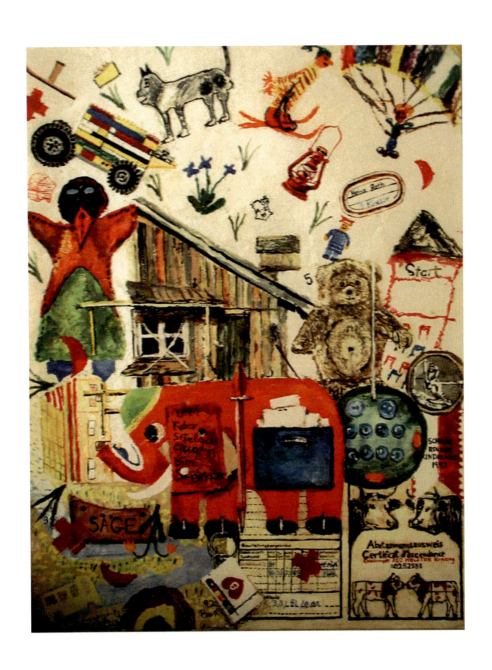

The son of a very gracious family in Grindelwald, paid me $20.00 to do this for him. His family showed me real grace.

A LOOK INSIDE THE MANIC:

Q
11
5
'J
r

Lady
with
Baguette
and
Poodle
in
France

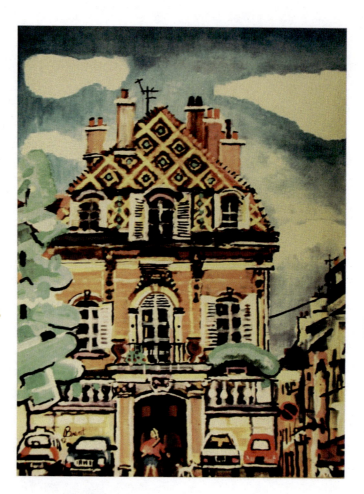

l ,.,vo.rI·1 .a.r...._r2 .c. =

o Id, pQin

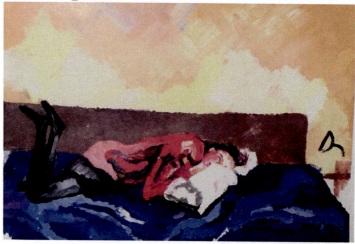

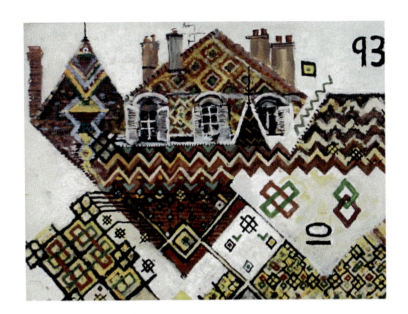

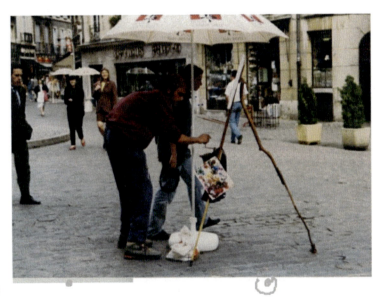

The stage of Dijon

III

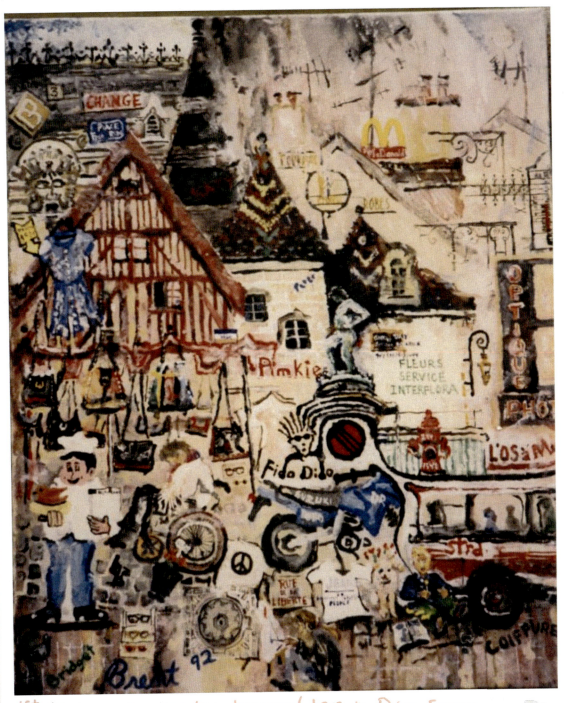

1st tears over a painting happened here in Dijon, France

- This painting sold in a contest/fundraiser. The French made painting magnificent.

de11eloped w..s" fif'll

COllS,,.,

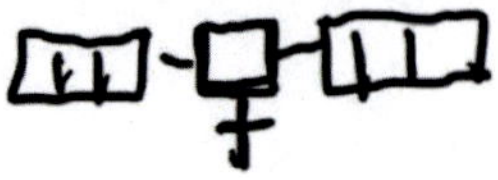

-pro,is,.

Back to the good ole

:t *f,J(;j   f'f 'ti4,j f'p ..,..,*

US of A

♩ *re5f-4vr411 psr*

JV) Ot\ -1-

and back to **G**

to finish Architecture Degree

~~I re+vrf\4!-d~~ returned

4! ro.n from
fu,-ope. ~~Europe tht~~
nkJ'''jr *and painted the Restaurant Series*

Thinking. I could.

l.o"ld pQi-.t- paint ltk.e
like tke..the

wind.

Re. e.,.beri"

Dropped out of G for 2nd time to paint *following my #/passion*

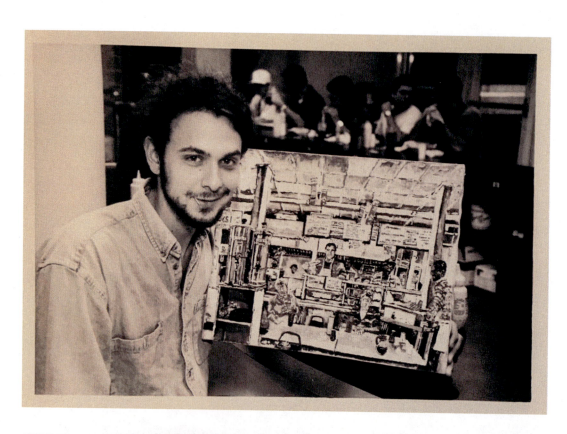

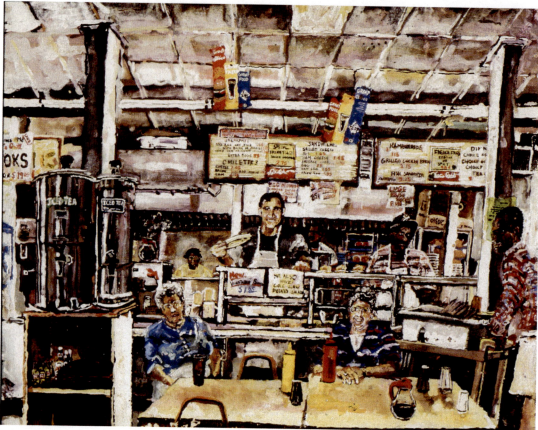

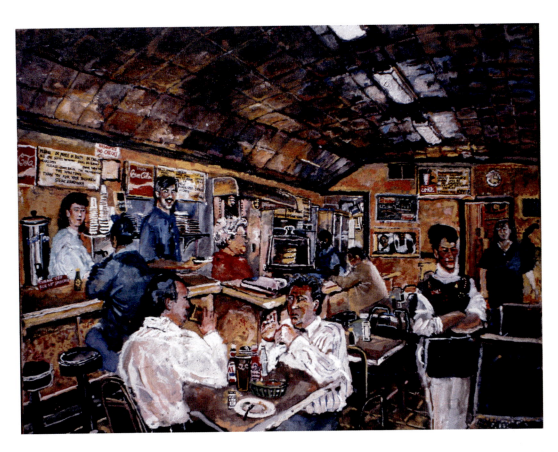

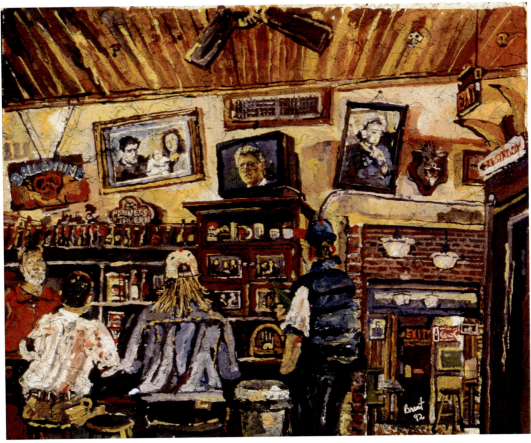

di -P"" /)J,)(0

H;.sRosewood aod Bfrdseye Maple paio, bo, isopeo ;o h;s, =m. Gouache p,;o,s **spread out.**

made at G

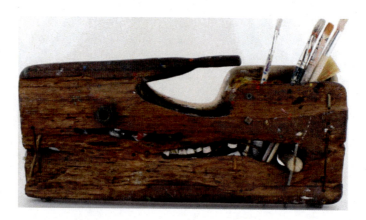

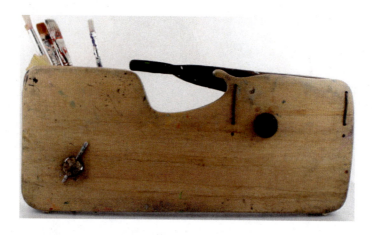

My paintcase I built, when I returned home from Europe.

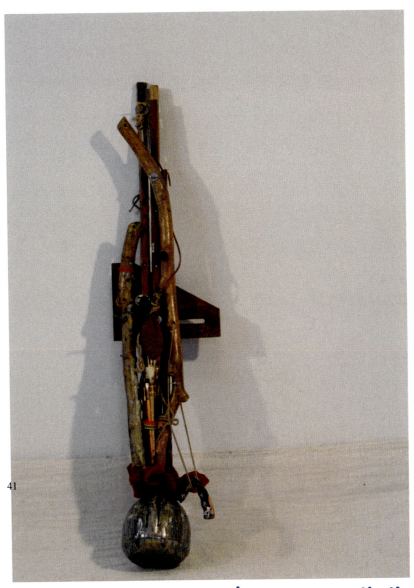

"shadow cello"

It takes about 15-20 minutes to set up in useable form... Time to switch from left to right brain & focus.

majestics

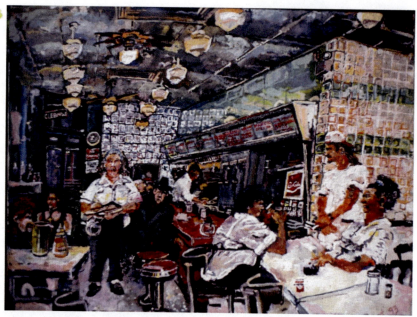

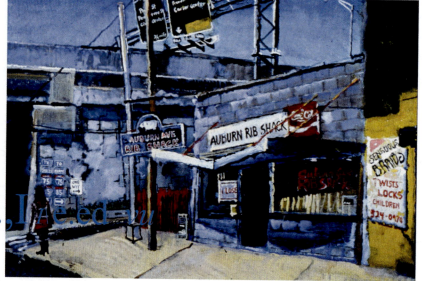

J.,I AC ed

Majestics was the official 1st in Restaurant Series. Man in black = World famous violinist

Brother Juniper's

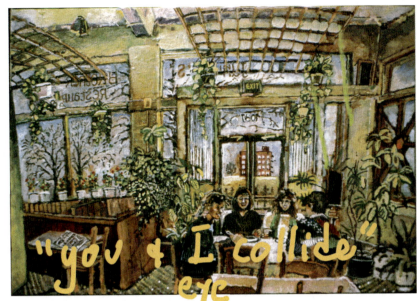

"you & I collide"
eye

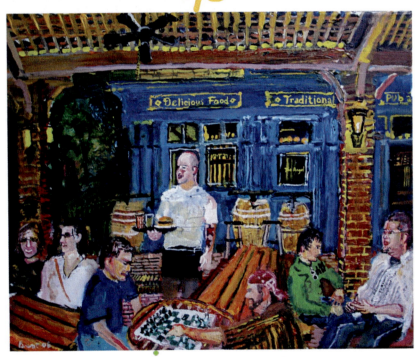

↑
me

New
Treasury Building, sits outside of windows where Brother Juniper's used to be.

Me and E had spent many a night drinking coffee around town.

One night we went to the Carlos Museum at Emory University. She pointed to some kind of fertility goddess, or wedding trinket. We were the only people I recall in the Museum, and I thought she was insinuating to me that she wanted to get married. I don't know if it was just the look in her eyes. It may have been how and what she said, in particular, about the object. This may be the very first sign of illness I can recall. I took her words as a hint of her secret thoughts about the two of us. WRONG! But, I have gotten way ahead of myself. I was becoming convinced that I was the one for her, even though we had not been "dating."

After the night at the Carlos Museum, I was working at E's mother's house. Relocating plants in the backyard was suppose to be an easy job, but I began seeing the plants as representations of people. One little tree I was asked to move, I saw as E herself. Its roots were wrapped around the roots of a larger tree. I argued not to move it. The tree would not survive chopping its roots up to free it from the larger tree. In my heart, it was to be protected.

Later at E's mom's house, I built a soldier out of the trash can just for the fun of it. There was a sword in one hand and a basket of flowers in the other.

The same day, I encircled another tree with stones. Why? I can not remember. E's mom also wanted me to chisel the tile out of the shower. I left the tiles forming a big horizontal E that kind of looked like a W.

The next morning, I went to North Georgia with my mom and dad. From the car, I started seeing black and white patterns. Things started to shift slowly. On the way home, I told Dad in the car, "I think someone is messing with my head!"

Dad showed concern, but did not say anything.
Mom made some statement about Satan and the mind.

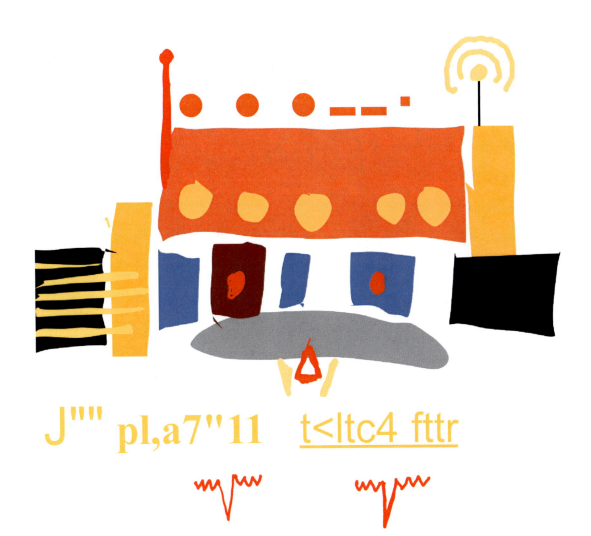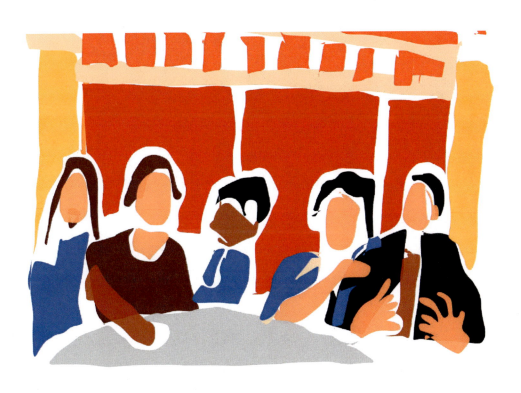

(?) Devil on

I was cocky, like Johnny

ending down deep I wanted to put an exclamation mark on Postmoder
Ism
Its over   His own and beat   Truth wins! & not just the Aim for truth
r-e   t-   t,er,...d c.,...Jct

then
The Devil went Down to Georgia)

the   Hmmm?

leCAf er

A LOOK INSIDE THE MANIC

To Escape Painting

I had a good lady friend named "E." In the year I had been home from my second year long trip to Europe. We had magically-shared times, spinning and laughing while rolling down the hill near the lake at Emory. We

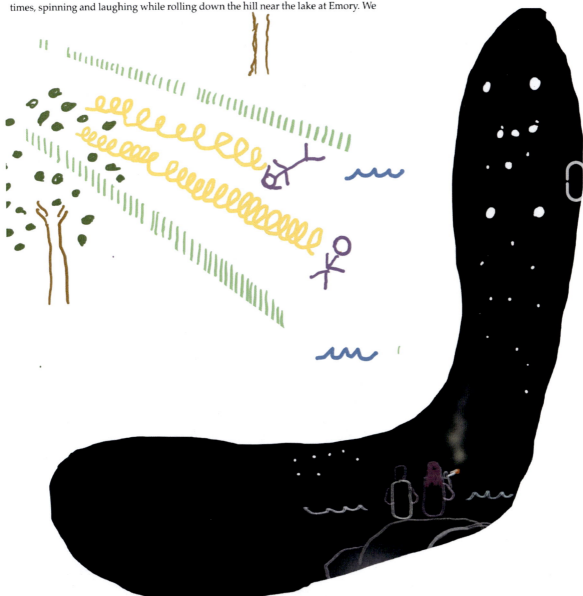

3. fllqnil Intrusion of rY\qtrr e

Assoc.1at,ons-

I walk past the ticket

[The INNOCENCE MISSION'S *Umbrella* CD is sof tly playing in the background.]

BRENT WRITES

I race into forever, beyond eternity
And still the SOUNDS persist. In heat,
Ram horns buck. Ram Horn. Earthqua ke divides
the two and one falls into the abyss.
Silence of b reat h as the fau l t separates
lo ne survivor from the herd. Feet tramp the
crevice looking for a point to cross.

Eerie
The
beside

There are sound s of very faint WEDDING BEL[...] Brent stops writing, looks out
at the da rknesses, and is perplexed. [Th ere is a s[...] the darkn esses fade into flashback.

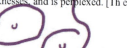

?

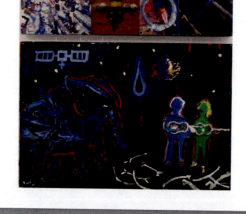

'94 - Things get weird, Fast!

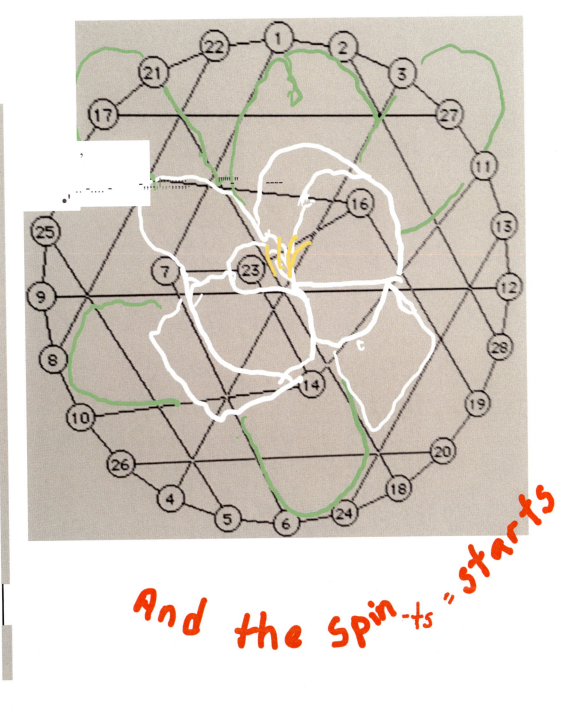

And the spin-ts = starts

EXT. DECATUR MARTA TRAIN STATION ----- DAY ————————FLASHBACK

Brent gets off th e MARTA train at the Decatur station. Brent is walking behind the statio n towa rds the buses . He sees a la rge pie ce o f an orange peel o n the ground. It is... a single peel spread out like a flowe r. He stops and stares.

> *BRENT (V O.) (remembering a quote from E)*
> "He wanted to watch a baseball game? Our ma rriage was already at a tenuous point, and he wouldn 't even go on a walk and share an orange. I knew then! Not long later, we were divorced."

Brent picks up the piece of ora nge and gently lays it back on the ground fee lin g e mp a thy for *E*.

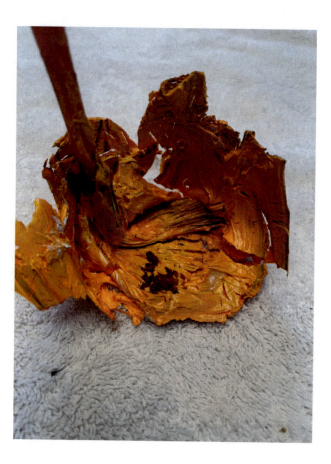

Story is starting

BRENT (V.O.)
I'd have taken that walk with her any day.

He continues walking towards the buses, and on a circular, iron sewer cap, he finds a fresh magnolia flower exactly centered. The geometry of the flower petals match the angles within the design of the sewer cap. It catches Brent's eye. He looks all around. The closest magnolia trees are very distant.

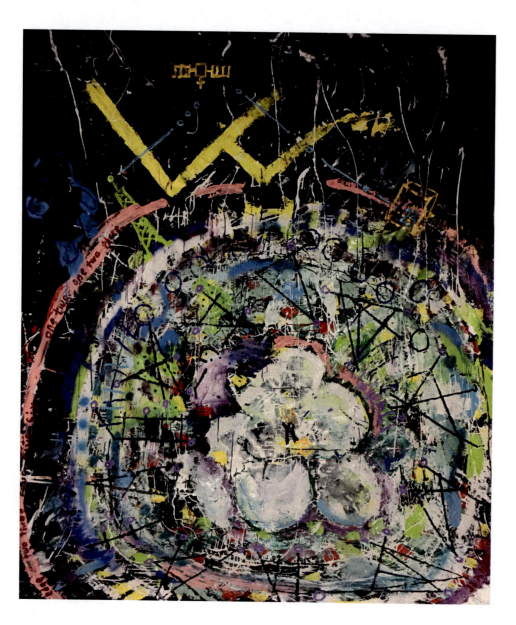

Painted 2018

This takes up a whole wall,

Brent appea rs pu zzled as he kneels down on one knee and takes a closer loo k. He checks the strength of the wind by lookin g at the overhead trees. The sun is bright and

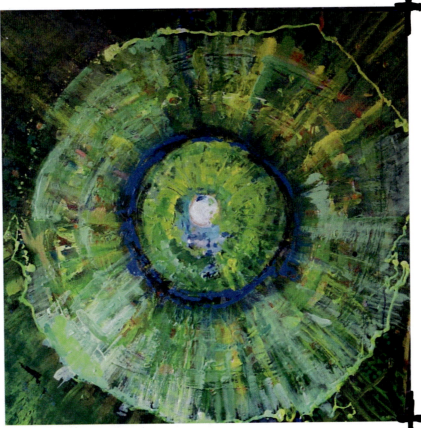

beaming through leaves th at are barely moving. A blackbird takes off from the top of a tree. It flies to a near by sidewa lk and picks some thing up. It flies away.

        BRENT
        Okay?

        BRENT *(V 0.)*
        Weird... not the wind. Someone must have placed that magnolia

Hmm?

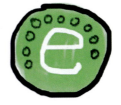

"elevation" unknown caller

I

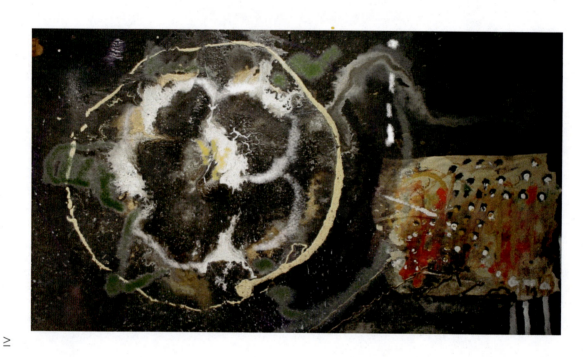

● is the path for me to her place.

●

He picks up the magnolia flower from the blackness of the iron.

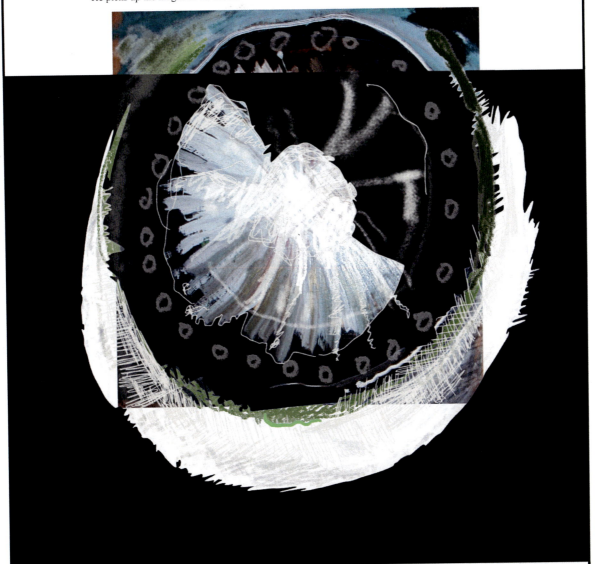

INT. E'S APARTMENT ------ NIGHT -----------<u>FLASHBACK</u>

Tt is very late at night. Brent is sitting on a loveseat with E.

BRENT

E, is this the loveseat that belonged to my parents *'j)*

This painting was actually done in response to Parsivel from the Holy Grail & his relationship to Blanche Flower

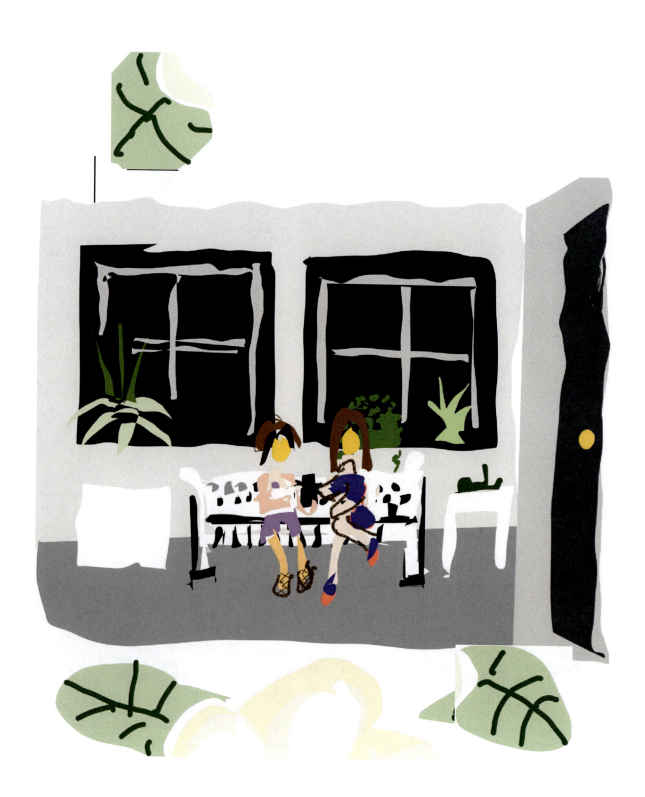

re-upholstered. How do you like the black and white check?

>BRENT
> I think it matches THAT.

Brent points to the low lit wall.

> E.

Yes, your mom gave it to my mom, and she gave it to me. I had it

> E.
> What?

> BRENT
> Did you do that drawing?

E nods, pleasantly shocked and surprised.

> BRENT *(seriously)*
> That's pretty cool. What does it mean to you?

Brent spots some lace used as decoration under the painting, and does not hear the answer.

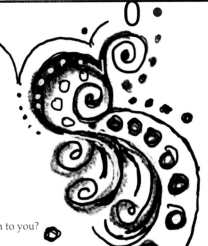

> BRENT
> Well, the swirls of the painting and the lace below look like a wedding or possibly a wedding dance.

> E.
> Like that! Pretty astute. Most people would not bring that interpretation.

E looks away. E gets up and gets her journal from a bookcase. When she returns she sits close to Brent. E is reading from her journal and showing him more black and white ink drawings. Brent doesn't hear E's words, except when a green drawing appears.

> E.
> How do you like the vines? Notice the lace pattern. I'm proud of this.

Brent tries to put his arm around E.

Oops

> E.
> Don't you think it is a little too early for that?

Brent pulls his arm back in an extremely awkward moment. They both then smile at each other.

> BRENT
> You know E, tonight it seemed when I was coming to your apartment that there were concentric rings, waves of energy, that seemed to get more intense the closer I got to here.

> E.
> I understand. Sometimes places and people give off particular energies. Nothing particularly uncommon about that.

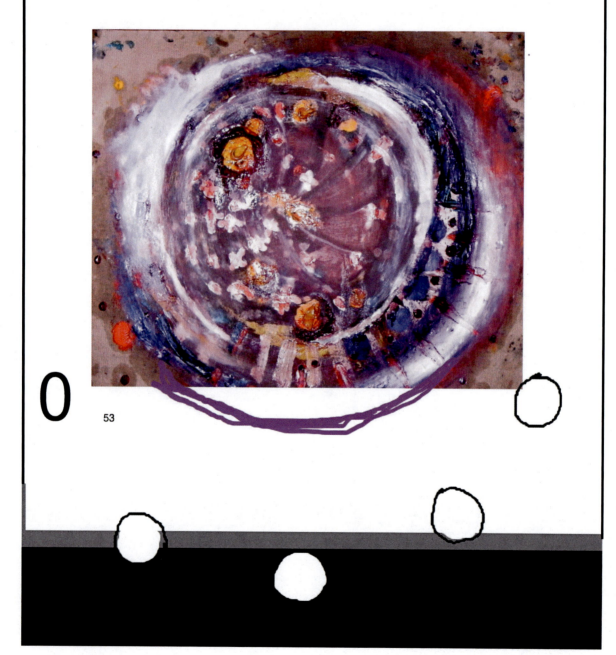

                                       Li
                                       N le   e \

      BRENT
      It is really getting late, maybe I should go.

      E.
      Yeah.

      BRENT
      See ya again sometime?

      E.
      Of course.

EXT. BACK at SEWER CAP WITH MAGNOLIA FLOWER -------------DAY

Brent holds the flower as someth i ng very preciou s.
[Focus on the white of the flo wer and blackne ss of the sewer cap.]

        BRENT (V 0.)
        Bride and Groom? We have not even really dated? Come on, admit
        to yourself you like her. You knew when you met her at home, she
        could be the one! Should I associate the flower with her
        black and white motif?

I NT. BRENT'S PARENT'S HOUSE ----- DAY ----- FLASHBACK   **O**   **u>**

Brent enters the living room of the house he grew up during high school. He has   **y,_**
recently gotten home from Europe and is full of confidence. He comes in talking, and
sees *E* sitting on the piano bench. She is facing the room instead of the piano. Brent's
mom is sitting in a chair. He shuts up immediately when he sees *E*. Brent had forgotten that his
mom wanted him to meet someone. He obviously is not expecting a gorgeous
woman wearing a strange, maroon, mushroom hat.

                                                                   ")

                                                                   f'

           Hey Brent, you remember I wanted you to meet someone. Do you

           remember *E* from DeKalb Christian Academy? Her brother was

           in   your class. She's pretty smart!   \ genius

r'

        E. (looking at Brent)
        Yeah, M, he's my brother. I was a few years ahead of you.

linguistic intentionality   J \ C,

u s

> BRENT *(staring at E, kind of stunned)*
> I love that HAT!
>
> E.
> Thanks!! I hear you were in Europe for a year painting on the streets. You must have some serious skills.
>
> BRENT
> Yeah! Where did you say you got that hat?

Brent look s at his mom. E's answer doesn't register. Tt was no place he had heard of.

> BRENT
> I've never seen one like that. You look great in it. So, just how do you know my mom?
>
> £. *(S miles)*
> Remember your mom and my mom are best friends. Your mother helped me after my divorce, and she got me through some of the deeper issues I was going through... *(conversation continues)*

EXT. DECATUR MARTA STATION ------------DAY

Brent, still holding the magnolia flo wer, realizes it's too hot out to carry it on the bus.

> BRENT *(V O.)*
> It won't make it to E's apartment. It will wilt.

He returns the flow e r to the sewer cap as he found it. Brent cont i nue s a lon g the path to the bu s, and not far from the mag nolia flo wer, he sees a piece of folded pap er in the downspout on a nearb y bu il di ng. He wa lks to the down spou t, pull s out the pape r, and opens it to find a li s t of so ngs, hand w ritten.

> BRENT *(V 0.)*
> Songs? This wouldn't be a list of songs for a wedding would it? Oh my God. I need to ask *E* what's going on here when I see her.

There are chalk draw ings on the pa vement. It looks like kid drawing s. Brent appears a tad anxious as he now thinks, for the firs t time, that these contain information. He is puzzled and soon forgets them. Now he starts picking up tiny pieces of paper . Candies and trash left outside , are all clues on the ground. He finds a business card for a

password: V Enter here   In your eyes

TATLOR that is advertising business concerning "Wedding Apparel."

>BRENT (V.0.)
>Damn! This is serious! I gotta know if, by chance, *E* wants to marry me.

Brent finds a telephone booth and calls the phone number on the tailor's business card.

>BRENT
>Hi, this is Brent Weston. Do you know anything about a wedding concerning *E?*

>TAILOR (in *a foreign accent*)
>I am afraid I cannot help you. Let me get *(Jan e Doe)*. Maybe she can help you.

>JANE DOE
>Hello?

>BRENT
>My name is Brent Weston. Are you working on a wedding dress for *E?*

>JANE DOE
>Can you repeat that please?

>BRENT
>My name is Brent Weston, and T think Tam supposed to be marrying *E*. I want to know if you are working on her dress.

>JANE DOE
>I not sure what you mean. I do not think I can help.

>BRENT
>Okay, I'm sorry.

Brent gets on the bus. The bus will only take him part way, and he has to walk a ways to E's place. She lives just off of Clairmont and North Druid Hills. While walking, *E* dr ives by. She stops the car and rolls down the window.

>E.
>Where have you been? You are over an hour late.

Brent jumps in the car.

INT BAKERY ------DAY

Looking through an outside window at a bakery, Brent and E are talking at a table on the inside. Their voices are silent. [Cut to the inside of the bakery.] Brent pulls out the change in his pocket. He has a round, metal washer amongst the coins. E gen tly takes it out of his hand.

> E.
> Curious, where did you get that?
>
> BRENT
> I found it along the road. Makes me feel lik e I have an extra penny in my pocket. You know I'm doing the poor artist gig right now. I'm too broke to even be in a relationship. Think I shoul d make that into a piece of jewelry? Possibly a ring?
>
> E.
> Maybe. I'm not sure what to do with it, but I understand the poor artist thing.

She has a secret Garden

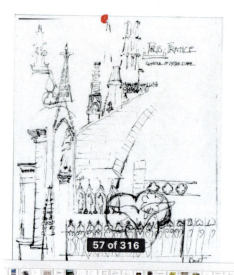

Holy Moly This morning I drew this page from a bad screenshot & Notre Dame caught fire in Paris. This sketch was from my traveling journal of ND.

E hands the washer back to Brent.

INT BACK AI BRENT'S ROOM ------NIGHT TIME

Brent is standing staring out the window at the darkenesses. [WEDDING BELLS, chime faintly... as if from an ancient European cathedral.] One of the neighbor's roosters crows three times around two o'clock in the morning . [It is much louder than the bells.]

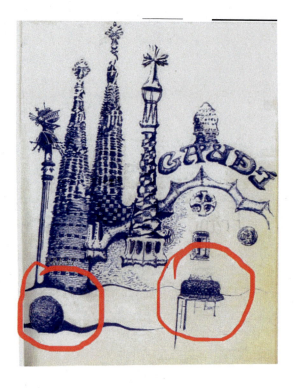

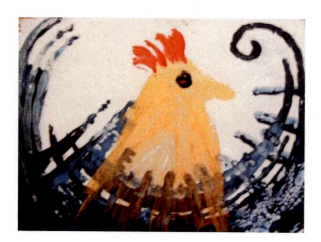

Damn Roosters! And bells! I should have had the moxie to ask her!

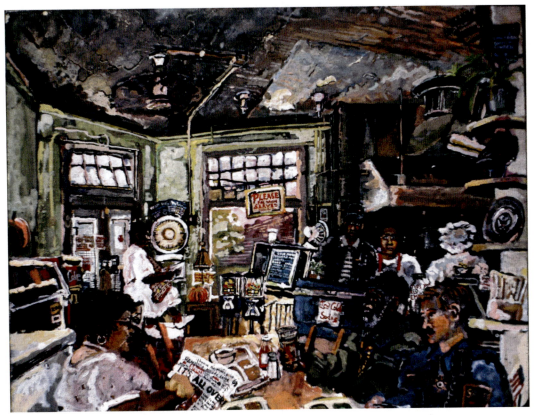

Deacon Burton's Grill

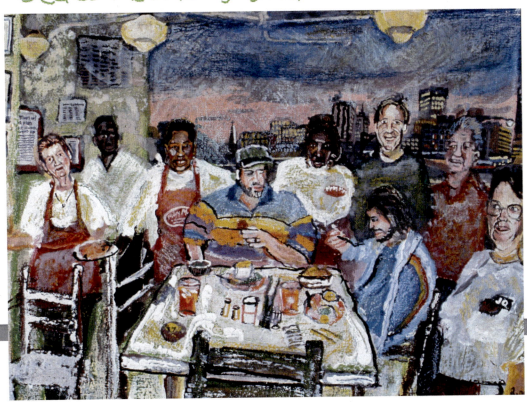

me d "T"

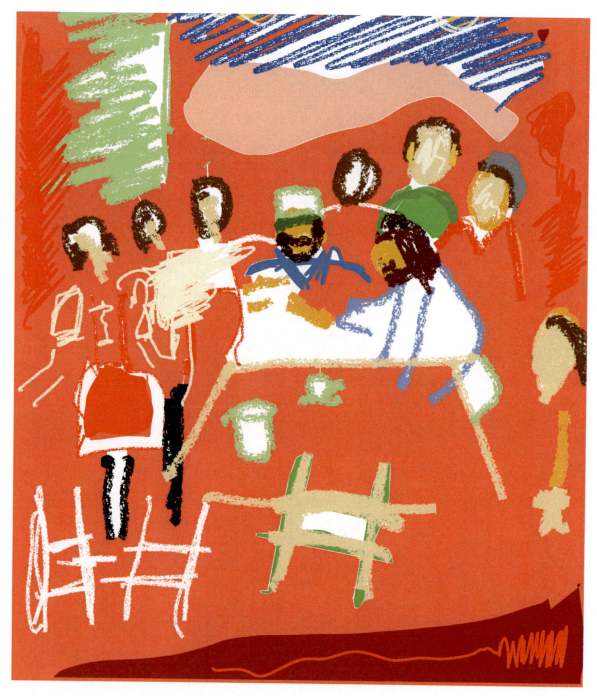

I have no money, but she may have this already planned out somehow. Bells. Those are original. Someone is having a church service at two in the morning? No way. This is bizarre. Could it be a wedding? No way! Not much has made sense today. It's *E,* it's gotta be. She doesn't always make sense. She thinks beyond me and sees what I don't. Is she calling me from the church up Moreland? God, she's the only one I'd marry. She IS smart enough to pull off all this. I just need the courage to show up!

    BRENT
    I love you *E.*

Brent looks at the paintings and their tiny details, forgetting about his Patron sponsored restaurant series.

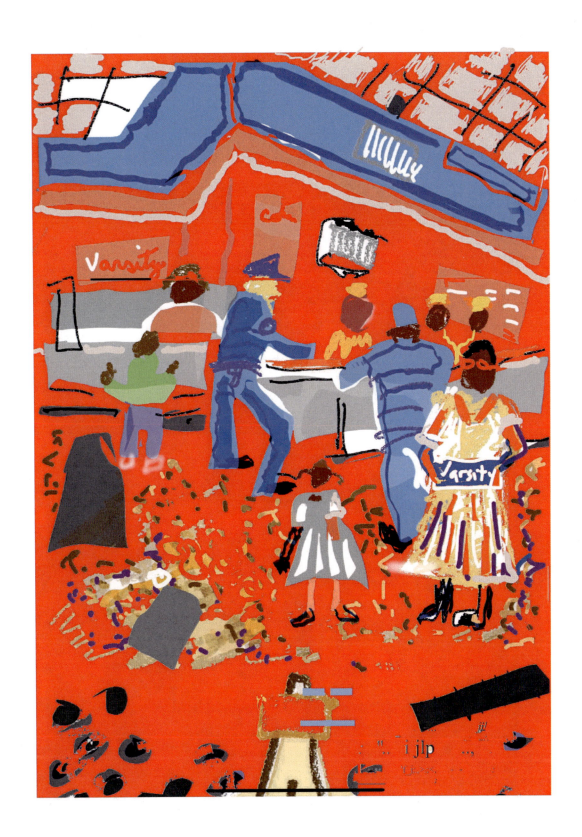

Thelma's

Thelma's fr\05, Kcrchen

Varsity

VGr.s.1

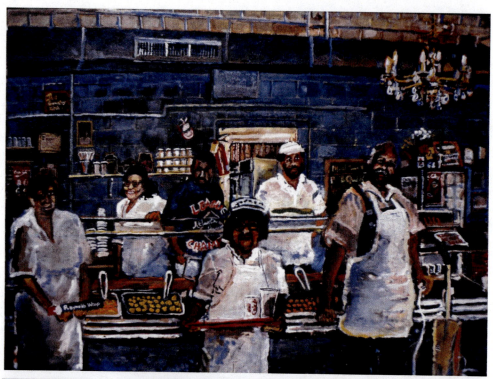

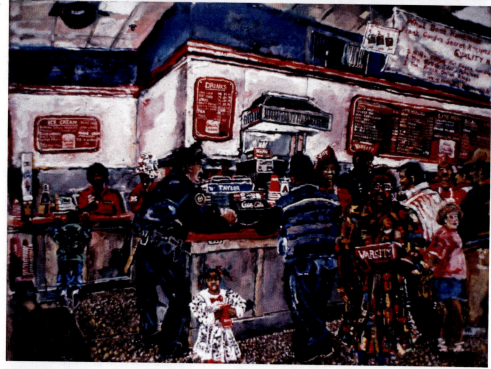

There were over twenty people watching me do a painting live of this lady

most pqimint dt> Alex's Barbeque Heaven

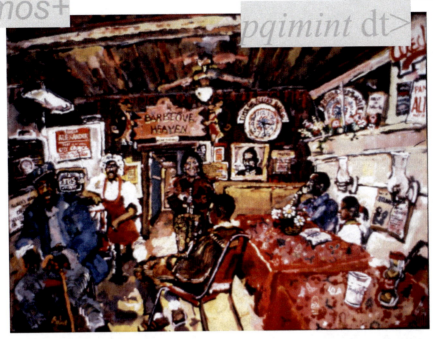

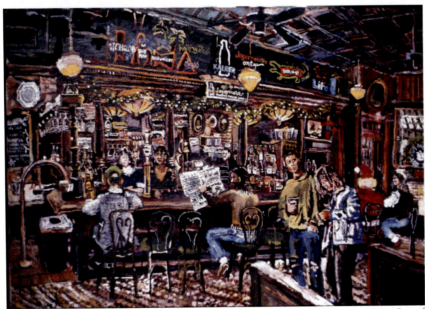

Atkin's Park Pub

wrl-helpo--P Ji

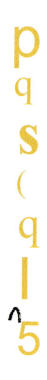

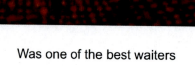

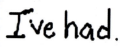

Was one of the best waiters

Rumors had it that some of the original bus strikes during the Civil Rights movement were originally planned at Pascal's Restaurant.

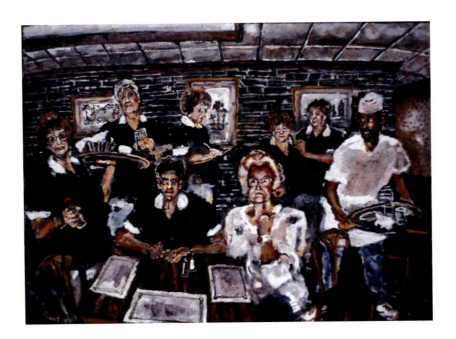

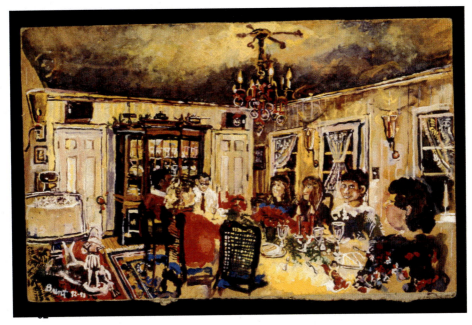

This Christmas painting is very "PC" Polish, Asian, African American...

> BRENT (V.O.)
> The bells? It is 2am; this is not happening. Is the wedding now!? I've got to know! I'm going down there to check!

He jumps up barefoot, journal in hand, to take a look. He is rushing with adrenalin. His hair is still disheveled.

EXT. BRENT'S RENTED HOUSE ---------NIGHT

As the bells continue to ring, Brent hurries out of the house, turns right, and runs down the street.

> BRENT (VO.)
> Could this be it! Oh my God. I cannot believe it. Goodbye virginity.

EXT. CHURCH ---------NIGHT

He stops in front of a yellow church. No one is there. There are bells ringing, but there are no church-bells on this church. He looks at the empty parking lot.

> BRENT
> Okay?

> BRENT (VO.)
> Shit, I am now confused. The wedding bells are real, but just a clue that I'm getting married? Or at least someone is.

The bells have now stopped ringing.

> BRENT
> I heard those bells! Where are y'all?

He turns left and walks, forgetting about the bells. He is still holding his journal in his left hand very tightly.

> BRENT (V.O.)
> Whatever the case, I can't wait to show *E* my poems.

EXT. GRANT PARK-----------NIGHT

A man on a mission, he walks down the si dewa lk scouring everything in sig ht for any d ues. He finds nothing out of the normal except some black charcoaled wood on the tip of a white, painted line in the parking lot. He interprets this as a long cigarette. He hears a human making a BIRD WHISTLE, coming from somewhere in the park.

> BRENT (V. 0 .)
> Bells? And now a human 's whistle? T! He's in my inner circle, and I trust him. He would definitely be at my wedding. He makes that whistle sound while goofing around. Of course! The park, a great place to get married. £! God, this is a big park.

A few homeless men glance his way -
Brent jogs through the park, past men on benches under newspapers - Bird whistles continue in the trees -
Halfway down a hill -
He trips, rolls the rest of the way dow n, and bounce s to a stop - No wedding party -
He catches his breath and sees part of a sign that says "ATLANTAZOO." He now hears chatter and a group singing in the distance.

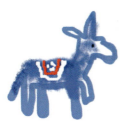

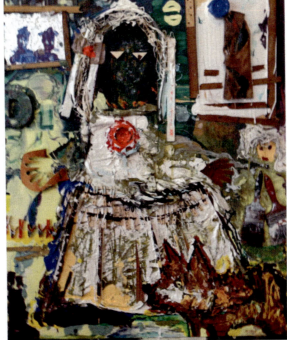

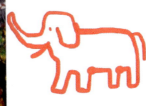

.--• e

> BRE NT (VO.)
> Interesting. *E* does like animals. Okay. Tf they are having a service in there, I AM curious. Plus, I am willing to get married in the zoo in the middle of the night, if she is. How do I get in?
> She IS creatively crazy, but I like it.

EXT. ZOO ---------NIGHT

Brent climbs easily over the front gate of the zoo with his journal. He wanders past elephants, zebras, and giraffes. He picks some flowers off a tree that is possibly a Magnolia. He squats in front of a black statue of an adult lioness and her cubs. He sets down his journal next to the lioness.

> BRENT (V O.)
> Hmmmm. How many children will we have?

Brent counts as he lays the flowers in a circle around the statue and sits down.

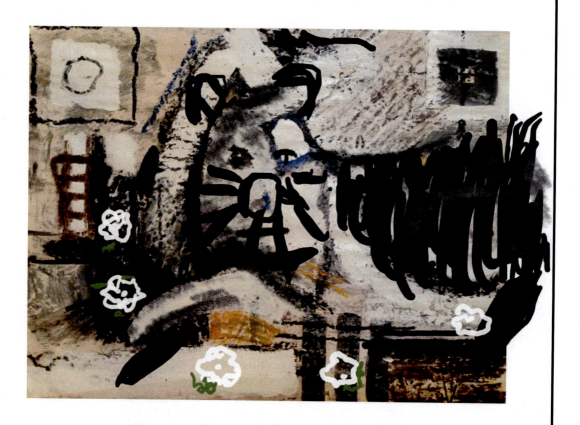

> BRENT (VO.)
> One. Two. Three. Four. Five. Yes, possibly five.

He grins slowly and laughs nervously.

> BRENT
> Five kids. I'll be a good dad if I can just sell some artwork.

He stands up.

> BRENT (VO.)
> No kids without the wedding first.

He resumes his wandering and pauses at the monkey cage. Their hands snag his attention. He looks at his own hands, and is surprised to find them empty.

> BRENT
> My journal!?

A SECURITY GUARD steps out of the shadows.

> SECURITY GUARD
> Can I help you!?

> BRENT
> Yes. Have you seen my fiancee?

> SECURITY GUARD
> Son, what are you talking about? What are you doing in here?

> BRENT
> I'm looking for my fiance, and I think I am gettin' married!

> SECURITY GUARD
> How did you get in here?

> BRENT
> I climbed the front fence.

> SECURITY GUARD
> Let's go for a walk.

BRENT

Okay? But I gotta go back and get my journal first.

SECURITY GUARD

No, you don't.

BRENT

'Course I do. It has over a year's worth of personal stuff in it, and some of my best poems. I know exactly where I left it.

SECURITY GUARD

I gotta escort you out of here.

BRENT

Well, when you find it, it's back by the black lion. Will you leave it at the ticket gate? Please? I'll stop back by tomorrow and get it later.

SECURITY GUARD

Okay. There are a lot of drugs in this neighborhood. What kind did you take?

BRENT

No, I have never had any drugs. Remember the journal!

The security guard unlocks the gate and escorts Brent out of the zoo. He looks at the fence and points to Grant Park.

SECURITY GUARD (laughing)

You should look for your fiance over there. I thought I heard bells a few minutes ago. They seemed to be coming from that direction.

BRENT

You heard them, too. I already looked there, no luck, but thanks though.

The security guard watches, stupefied, as Brent shuffles through the parking lot. The security guard walks back inside the zoo locking the gate firmly behind him.

Over the years, this is the first of about 5 journals I have lost.

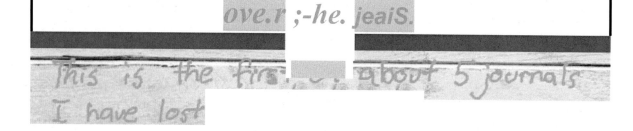

EXT. ZOO PARKING LOT ----------NIGHT

Brent s tops beside the two nice cars parked in the zoo parking lot. One is black; one is whit e.

> BRENT (V.O.)
> Wedding presents? They could have hid them better. I'll take them, though . Black an d white. I get the black one. No, no, no, no, no. E can pick first. Wonder where the keys are?

He searches under and around th e cars for the keys. No luck.

> BRENT (V.O.)
> I don't ge t it, Lord .

EXT. GRANT PARK------------NIGHT

Brent wand ers back through the par k and sits on a ben ch beside an OLD MAN .

> BRENT
> Have you seen a wedding party around here?

> OLDMAN
> What is the bride's name?

> BRE NT
> E.

> OLDMAN
> E? Nope. Haven' t seen E.

> BRE NT
> Thank s.

Br ent approac hes a MEXICAN LADY wit h a newspaper. She is w andering the park, too.

> BRENT
> Have you seen a wedding party?

> MEXICAN LADY
> Buenas noches.

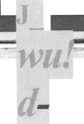
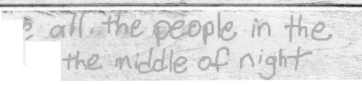

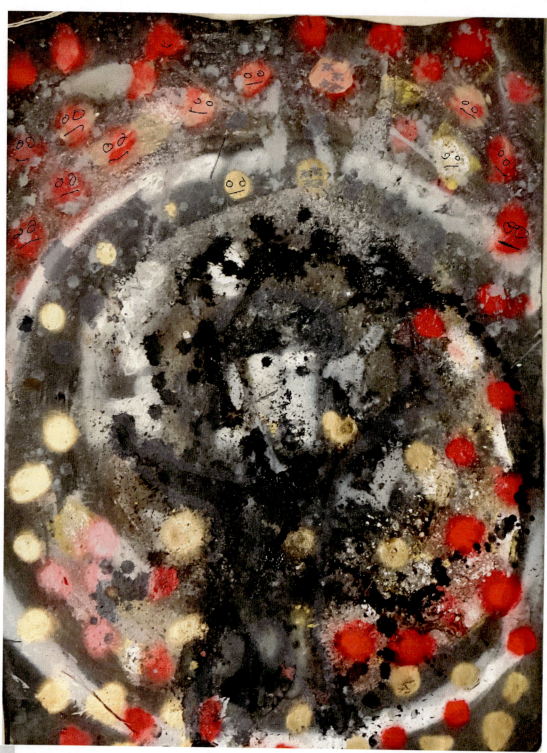

lah

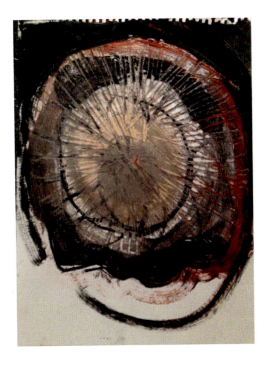

>   *BRENT*
>   Have you seen my fiance?
>
>   *MEXICAN LADY*
>   Olah.
>
>   *BRENT*
>   Olah?
>
>   *M E XTCAN LA DY*
>   Si!

She gives him the comics section of her newspaper.

>   *BRENT*
>   Is this for me? Are there clues in here that will tell me where the

> wedd ing is to be?
>
> MEXICAN LADY
> Si. Si.
>
> BRENT
> Excellent! Gracias!

The lady smiles. Brent walks away trying to decipher the comics; howe ver, he is hardl y able to concentrate.

> BRENT (VO.)
> This is confusing, and no clues are in here. Nothing but riddles.

He drops the comics to the ground and goes to the public tern-us cour ts. He invents his own game with objects placed on the court. It is as if, within the grid of the court, there are geometric hotspots that he is trying to find. Later , he sees a hubcap on the ground, picks it up, and carries it back home .

INT. BRENT'S HOUSE ····· EARLY MORNING

It is dark outside, and one of Brent 's ROOMMATES is still awake.

> BRENT
> I'll trade you tlus hubcap for information on where I can get my fiance an inexpensive but creative wedding ring. I'm kind of in a hurry.
>
> ROOMMATE
> How about Little Five Points. Who you marrying?

Brent gives him the hubcap.

> BRENT
> Thank you. Why did I not think about that?
>
> ROOMMATE
> What the hell is the hubcap for?

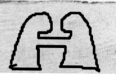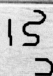

BRENT
There is something huge going on. Just remember the circle is a sign of infinite unity, like a ring. Any particular shop in Little Five?

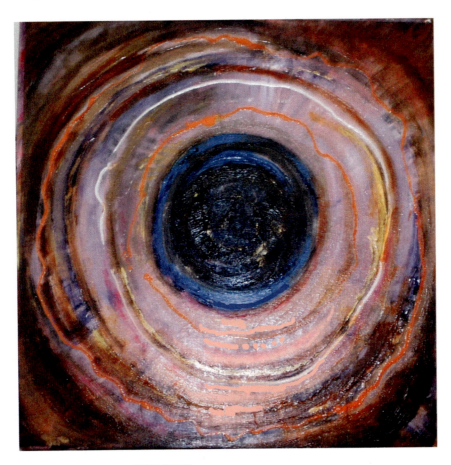

ROOMMATE
There are plenty of shop s, but they aren't open now. When you do go, be sure to get it large enough to fit her finger.

>BRENT
>Good info.

>ROOMMATE
>Who ya marrin'?

>BRENT
>It is a long story.

>ROOMMATE
>Ts this a 'b i g e vent ," or you e lo pi ng?

>BRENT
>Honestly, I am a littl e confused about the whole thing myself.

EXT. GRANT PARK------------SUNRISE

Brent exit s his house and walks back to the street exhausted, hopeless.
[DEPECHE MODE'S *Higher Love* is pl aying on his CD.]

>BRENT (V.O.)
>I am tired. Where are y'all? I'm about done looking.

A RUNN ER, dr essed in black and white, spri nts past Brent, dog in tow. His full face is hidden, but his visible lips move .

>RUNNER
>Stone Mountain.

>BRENT (VO.)
>Why did that runner say th at and keep on runnin g? The moun tain is a lo ng way fro m here. Stone Mountain would be the perfect place! The tip-top of the mountain. We both have good memories there. We have climbed it many times.

He looks down at his dirt y fee t.

>BRENT (V.O.)
>Must get sandals.

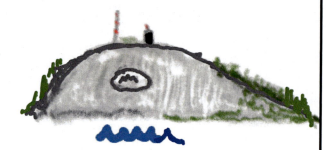

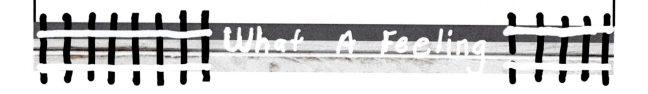

INT. PUBLIC BUS ---------DAY

Brent is now wearing his Jes us-loo king river sandals, plaid cotton shorts, and a thin white tank top that says "Hydra Greece " under a purple octopus wearing sunglasses.
He has his Georgia Tech backpack, some food, his Bibl e, and a Swiss Army knif e . He sits in the front of a bu s. A woman in a black and white suit is first to get on the bus. Brent briefly stares at the woman, pu zzled.

> BRENT (VO.)
> Half the city is involved in helping me get to our wedding ?

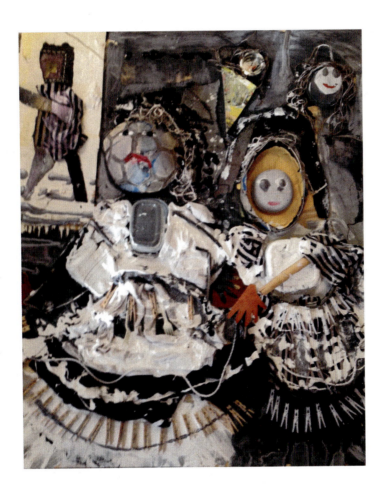

ThiS was cι. lo*bl.J.s* rtll., remembe J,!/f-le..

rhis *WAS* °" **IOI\:]** bus **rid4!**
i ɪ\ ,-.} **I\ı ch** . **r.** _{in which I} Little
remem be.r 1,=tf Je.

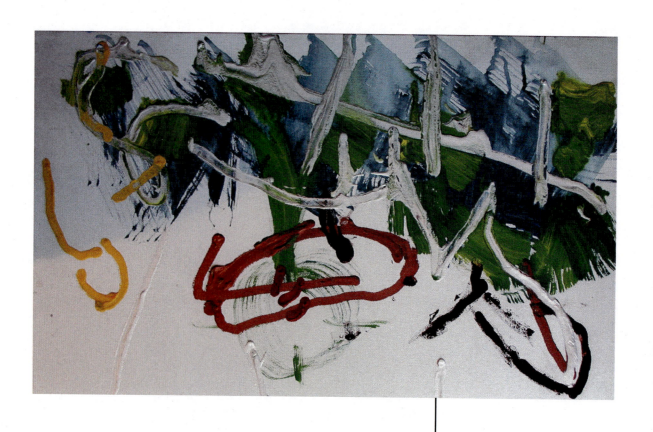

4. Pushing High up the Rock of Stone Mountain

EXT. BASE OF STONE MOUNTAIN ------------DAY

Brent kneels down in front of a black and white sign at the base of the mountain. He arranges several rocks in the shape of an "E," then removes some chicken from his backpack and places it amongst the "E."

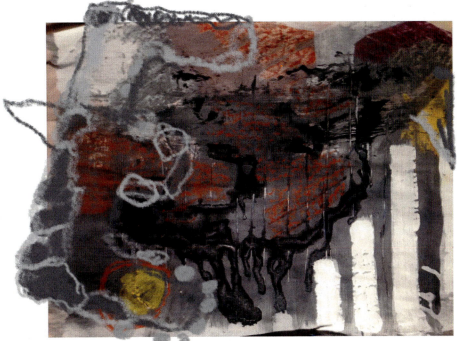

BRENT (V.O.)
E, are you "chicken?" He

starts up the mountain.

EXT. TRAIL UP THE MOUNTAIN ----- DAY

Along the way, he sees a bong on the ground; Brent has never done illegal drugs. He removes some grapes from his backpack and sh1ffs them in the bong. He also sticks a

74

:t.,-,..*4*,,..*11*   .. te   , **3rcr.pe.**
             1   -Po.
eo--i 11 10".   **Grapes/communion**

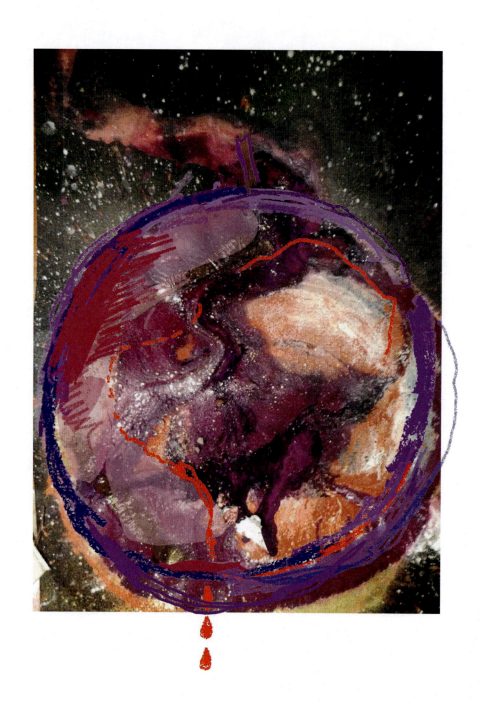

large log, at an upward angel, in the brick grill halfway up the mountain. He starts to feel dizzy in the heat of the sun.

> BRENT (VO.)
> I am going to make it. E, just give me a little more time.

He continues on and goes off the path into the shade of some trees. He pauses to pull out his small NIV Bible. He sits, hidden away from the path, to rest. He sees a very little bush/ plant, with fire red and orange leaves. He thinks they are discolored for this time of year. He makes a small crown of thorns out of sticks and lays it on the ground. The
leaves that had already fallen off the bush are poked onto the thorns. A breeze soothes his sweaty face. He opens the Bible to Ezekiel and skims verses already underlined.

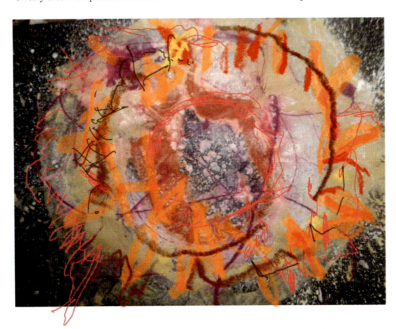

> BRENT (V.O .)
> Lord, where I go, I see patterns that involve people. A lot of people, all across the city! The patterns are also tied to a marriage motif. Is this going to be a wedding as large as an Old Testament story?

Immediately, a dove lands on a low branch two feet above Brent's head. Her feet are still as she scouts the territory. She walks to her nest a little ways down the branch. Brent is close to tears watching the dove within her nest, five feet from him. The timing to his question seems too synchronistic. He goes on to read prophetic words from Ezekiel, and Psalms 22.

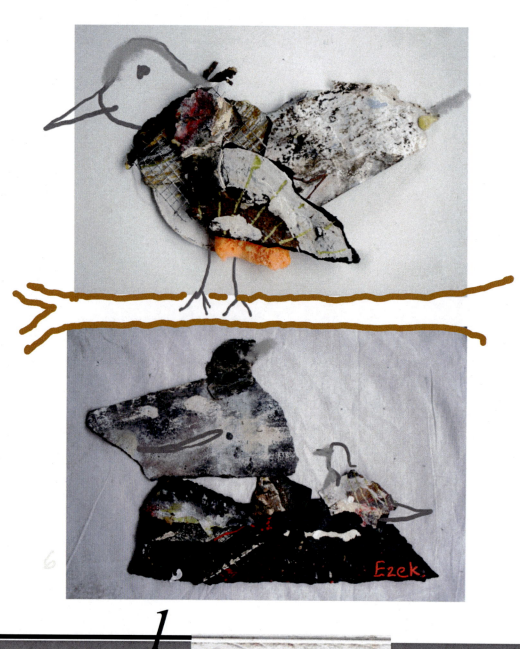

1

did cry.

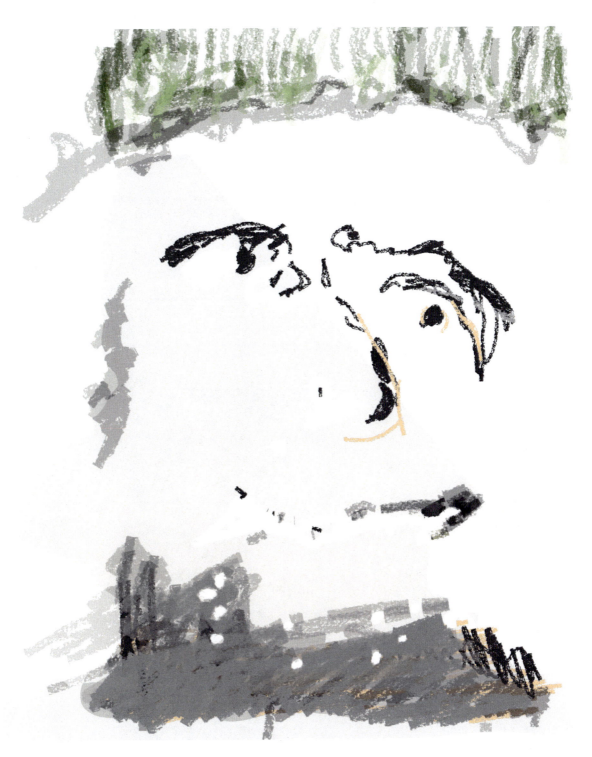

Aft e r a lon g rest, he continues on up the mounta i n. He hears an airplane and feels like the a i rpl ane is hovering overhead. He loo ks up a t an airplane in the sky, searching for its flight path to Hartsfield International Airport.

                BRENT (V O.)
       The day will come when they have technology to see me from up there.
       If this is as huge as I think, my privacy will be gone. No reason to hide;
       it would not work anyway.

Brent continues up the mountain. He pauses before a rock. There is a large face carved into the rock. THREE KIDS watch as Brent puts green sod on top of the rock's "head" and a cigarette butt in its "mouth." The kids just see a textured rock and not the face. The parents see the face.

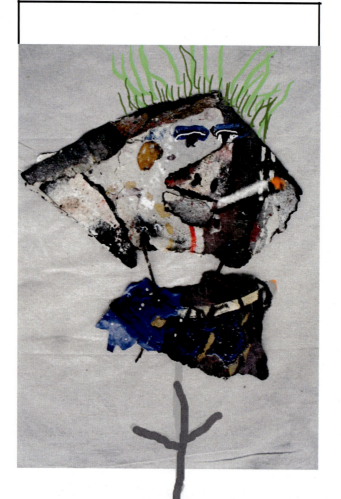

> KTDS
> What are you doing?

> BRENT
> I'm giving him green hair.

The parents point out the face, and the kids run off laughing.

> PARENTS
> Why did you put a cigarette in his mouth?

Brent does not answer, feeling somewhat ashamed.

EXT. MOUNTAINTOP ----------DAY

As Brent reaches the top, he feels an overwhelming sense of white and yellow from the sun, as if the light has penetrated and gone right through him. He looks at his own body, and it seems a transparent bright yellow. He blanks for a minute, and then crawls under the guard rail fence. He tosses the rest of his chicken over the side of the half dome, granite mountain.

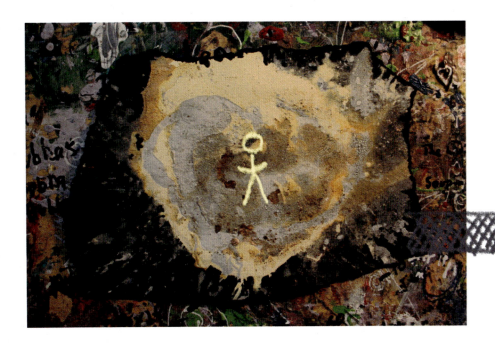

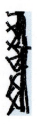

1043' above sea level

eaves the chicken. On that side
the fence and walks across the to

l

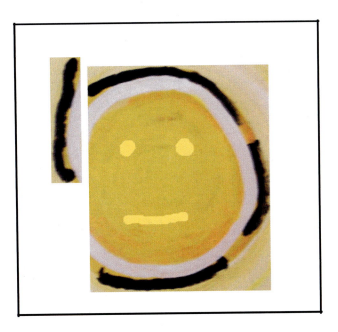

He s tagger s when he h He   of the fe nce, if he fa lls, he d ie s .
crawls back under   p. Still no we ddin g par ty.

        BRE N T (V O.)   t

        For the first time, I feel something really evil. Something IS evil here.

He sees strange words written in house paint directly on the granite. It talks weirdly
abouta cross.   /\

        BRE NT (VO.) .
        Is this where the KKK used to burn crosses? Maybe it is some pagan
        ceremonial place. I'm picking up bad vibes.

I \

Ye

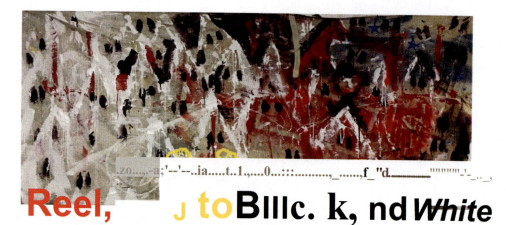

.zo......a;'--'--.ia....t..1.,...0..::...........,......,f_"d............""""""'-'-..-.,

Reel, ⌐ to Blllc. k, nd White
th1?yare precJou1 (precious) ,n (in)
His
S,9hT (sight)

EXT. MOUNTAINTOP BUILDING ----· DAY

After wandering in and around the architecture at the top of the moonlike mountain, Brent props open a lower, unused door. He builds a large sculpture in the middle. It looks like a military tank to him. He throws some M&M's he found on the ground, in the trajectory of the turret. He leaves the sculpture and approaches a lone, desolate, glass tower, which sits on the back edge of the mountain. People come and go in the adjacent buildings while the tower is locked. He wanders around the back.

EXT. GLASS TOWER   DAY

The glass radio tower has caught Brent's eye. It is five to six stories. Brent steps closer and sees a broken window at knee level. The original window frame is very large. The broken section is a vertical slit about 9 inches across and 2 feet high. Other vertical cracks surround the opening. [We see an abstract vagina in the opening and surrounding cracks.] Torn black paper flutters off parts of the edges of glass. Brent sits in front of the opening for an extra long time.

"But not only there; let freedom ring from the Stone Mountain of Ga."

> BRENT (VO.)
>
> *The Fountainhead* - Roark finishes breaking a marble fire place mantelpiece that Dominique had purposefully scratched. Doesn't Roark end up raping Dominique in the book not long afterwards? I am not Roark. Lord, help me here. I'm a virgin. If I go through that glass, am I metaphorically raping someone? E's not a virgin. This is going to be a metaphorical loss of my virginity. What would *E* want? WHY am I even thinking this way? Maybe E is saying I need to go through to get to the wedding. This is MESSED UP! I am going up to the helicopter! This is also the chance to see and go beyond the dark glass.

[There is a very faint HELICOPTER noise.]

A clean cut, middle-aged MAN IN A WHEEL CHAIR, rolls up beside Brent. Brent looks at him and thinks that he looks like a decorated war veteran.

> MAN IN A WHEEL CHAIR
> Are you thinking what I am thinking?

> BRENT (VO.)
> You want to get in there too, don't you?

> BRENT
> Would you go through that window if you could?

Man in wheel chair does not answer.

> BRENT (V.O.)
> You can't, but I can. In fact, I could do it for you.

Brent picks at the broken glass. He slowly wiggles a large section out of the frame.

> MAN IN WHEEL CHAIR
> That is some pretty sharp stuff.

> BRENT
> I will be careful.

Brent gently removes more broken glass from the large frame. The man looks at him and wheels away.

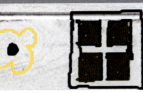
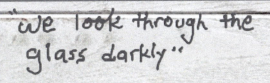

"we look through the glass darkly"

MAN TN WHEEL CHATR *(mutt erin g)*
Where's responsibility these days.

Brent notices the man wheel off.

BRENT (V O.)
It must be difficult for a wheel chair on the mountain.

He continues his work, quite good indeed, with the glass. [The helicopter noise slowl y grows.]

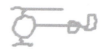

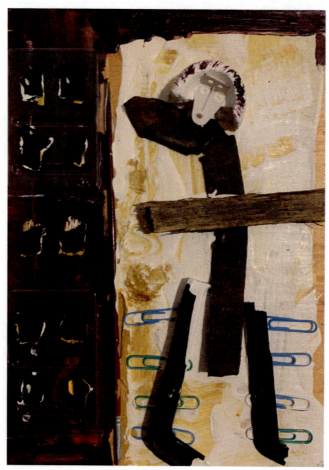

82

Thi! is acf v'1 ll1q porin-½ 1 o+'
-th O'\G\mber\itA -f?.ro

L1:1s /'Yle11Me.tS. 1 + Jvs-f nun;"r:J s-

This is actually a painting of the chamberlain from *Las Meninas* by Diego Velazquez.

It reminded me of entering in the tower

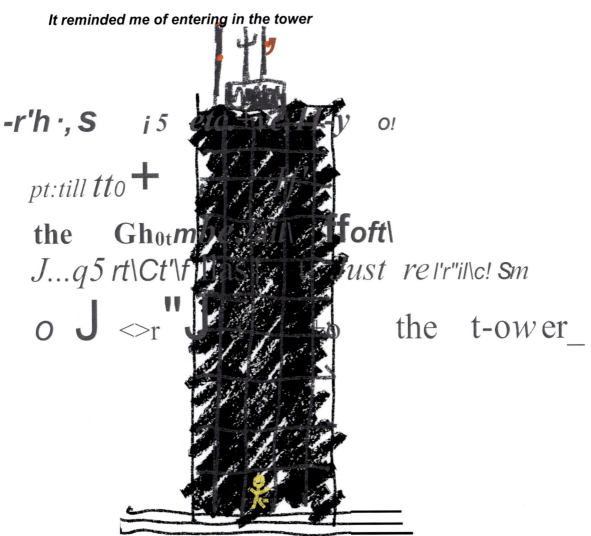

                    BRENT
          I'm coming! Just give me a minute to get up to the top of the
          tower.

[Pan the top of the tower and the sky around it.] There is no helicopter, only a bird soaring in the currents. Brent removes enough glass and PREPARES to go in.

                    BRENT (VO.)
          Well! Who else can say they got picked up by a helicopter to go to their
          wedding?

[The helicopter noise steadily grows louder.] He looks left, feeling the stare of POLICEMAN #1, who stands around the corner looking at him through the glass.

                    BRENT (VO.)
          Why are you not stopping me?

Policeman #1 doesn't move.

                    BRENT (VO.)
          Cool. Thanks for understanding.

Brent looks again at the policeman. He slowly lifts his left leg over a low pane of glass. The policeman sees him enter the glass tower. Their eyes meet. The policeman walks off. As Brent's foot touches down inside the tower, everything goes BRIGHT WHITE.

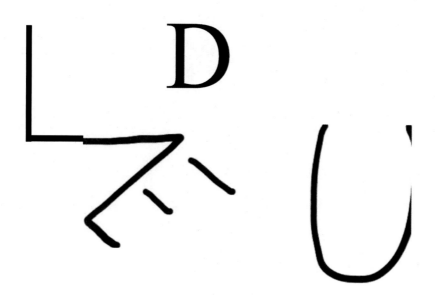

One time I was doing a painting based on this experience, on a glass door. As I was breaking the glass in the door, for therapy,... Pink Floyd's helicopter beginning started on radio.

!crec.'" weu

> BRENT *(Screaming, crying as loud as one can)* E! E!
> *E!* I'm here! I'm here!

[Slowly, the white dissolves.] Brent reappears, now standing inside the tower. His hair is dbheveled, his face swollen with tears. He stares up the inside steps that lead to the top. He is still crying.

> BRENT (VO.)
> Is intellectual intercourse before marriage really okay? It doesn't feel right to me. YET... E, has me for life.

> BRENT
> E! E! E! I LOVE YOU!

His gaze falls on equipment in the corner of the towe r. [Its volume meter rises and falls with Brent's voice.]

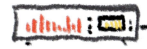

> BRENT (V.O.)
> The y're broadcasting me live on the radio. This has gone too far.

> BRENT *(yelling)*
> This is too personal!

EXT. TOWER ----------DAY

Policeman #1 and #2 run toward the tower.

INT. TOWER -----------DAY

Brent races up the stair s hearing the helicopter. At the top is a room. He is met with a lock ed, s torm-gla ss door attached to a huge plank of black, painted wood.

> BRENT (VO.)
> More glass?

> BRENT
> I'm almost there! Keep waiting!

The glass door is intact. He tries gently taking the door off it s hinges with his Swbs Army Knife. That does not work. He starts to unscrew the frame holding the door to

TM. /b'j hfl.lc£ t\o•he.

The **Voice** like the intensity of at a U2 concert.

the wood. [There are footsteps and voices at the bottom of the tower.] Brent freezes. He looks at the men in blue. Brent panics. Hemmed in, he puts his Jesus-saled foot through the glass. It shatters into fine beads. The wood plank does not budge.

> BRENT
> Come on. Come on.

> BRENT (V O.)
> This looks like a stage set up. No reason for a storm door on a flat piece of wood... and the way it broke?

He bangs his foot against the wood again and again, to no avail. The policemen reach the top of the stairs, guns drawn.

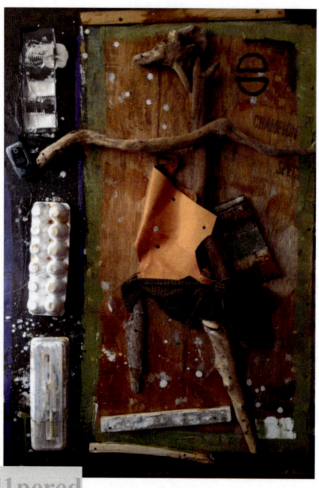

Tefl1pered

Glass?

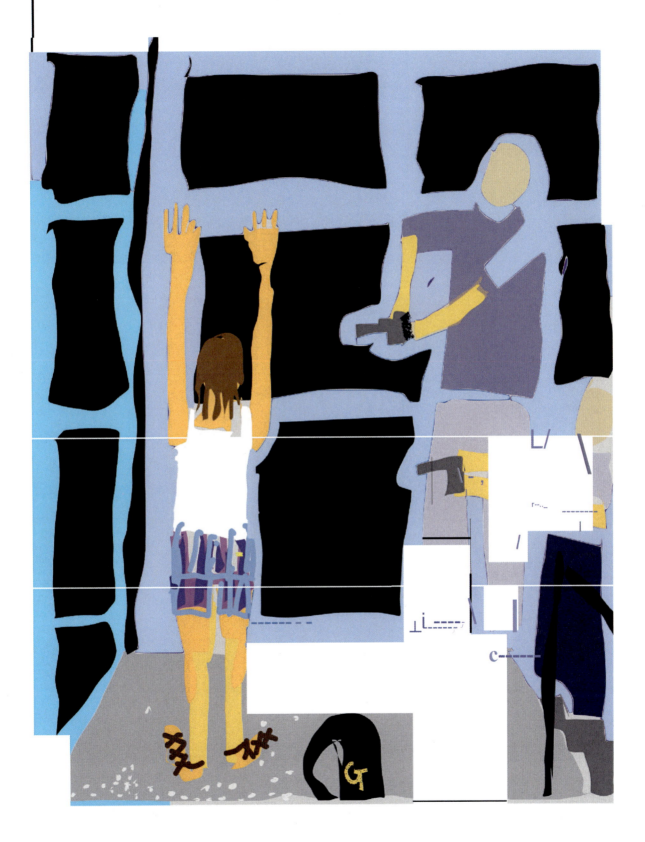

PO LTC EM AN # 1

FREEZE! Put your hands in the air!

Brent freezes, and puts his hands up.

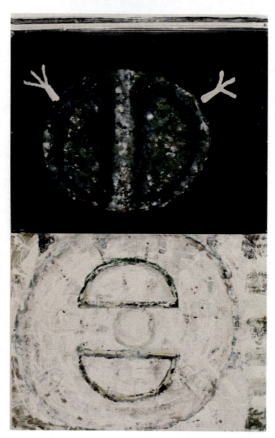

And if the mountains should crumble and disappear into the C, not a tear, no not I

I luv this painting ♥

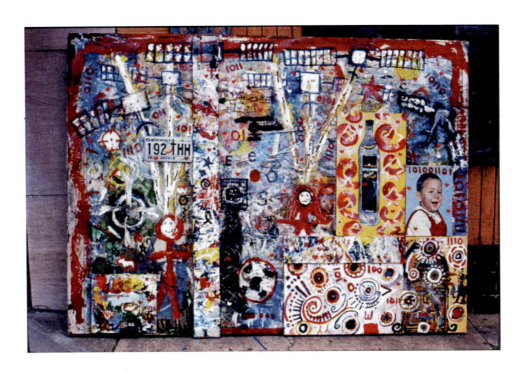

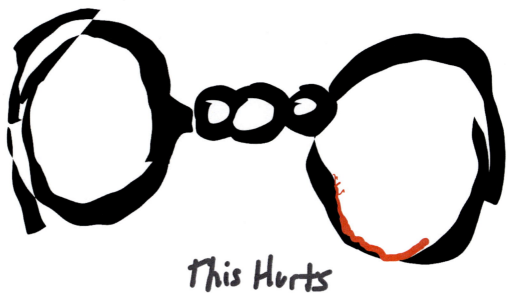

This Hurts

Postmodernism makes me laugh = True.
Postmodernism makes me cry.   =.True
Postmodernism offers no "intent"
to the universe. I think it says there
is no prime mover or no creator. BUT, it uses
intent to make its claim about itself. No one
can live consistently without some intent.

Policeman #2 opens up his handcuffs. Brent offers his hands without any resistance.

> BRENT (VO.)
> E/ I am here for you!

As he is cuffed, he looks down at the sparkling glass beads on the floor.

BRENT
Isn't that beautiful!?

POLICEMAN #1
Is what beautiful?

BRENT
Any of those would make the perfect ring for E. I don't think she would mind glass instead of a diamond.

POLICEMAN #2
You have a lot to figure out, son.

POLICEMAN #1
You have the right to remain silent. Anything you say ...

EXT. MOUNTAINTOP ---------DAY

They escort Brent past an extra long line of people who are waiting for the gondola down the mountain. Brent rides down the mountain with only the two policemen.

POLICEMAN #2
Do you understand your rights?

BRENT (completely seriously)
No. I- I -no - could you repeat them please? I'm not quite sure what's going on here.

5. Not Slee in as q JC4ilbird

INT. DEKALB COUNY CO TROOM---------DAY

[People fill half of the courtroom space.]
The policemen walk Brent in. Brent looks around excitedly.

BRENT (v.O.)
All you folks wanted to help me find the wedding! And you were all willing to break a few rules too, weren't ya! E's mom is rich; she's probably got over a million dollars.

Brent raises his voice.

The gondola ride seemed to last forever

> *BRENT*
> Hey everybo dy! I know someone who will pay our bail bon ds.

> *POLICEMAN # 1*
> Hush!

> *JUDGE*
> Order.

rieAce£

> *BRENT*
> She's lo aded. She will help us ALL out.

> *POLICEMAN # 2*
> Be quiet.

> *BRENT*
> I know you all are trying to help me. Even the police are in on it.

> *JUDGE*
> You, young man, are in contempt of my court. Get him out of the courtroom.

The police lead him out. Brent's eyes linger on an overhead light in the courtroom. [The light' s inten sity grows.] Behind the light, he sees himself and *E* holdin g hands. They are clothed only in light. He's mesmerized in a kind of afterglo w. He does not remember exiting the court room. The policemen haul him out into the atrium. Brent notices cameras for the first time in the corners of th e ceiling.

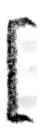 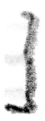

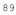

n,q{/11t::t''''c:,,.+ion j
vis ton

t c
h
e l
 o
 s
 e
 r
 . f

one.

ce,

P.

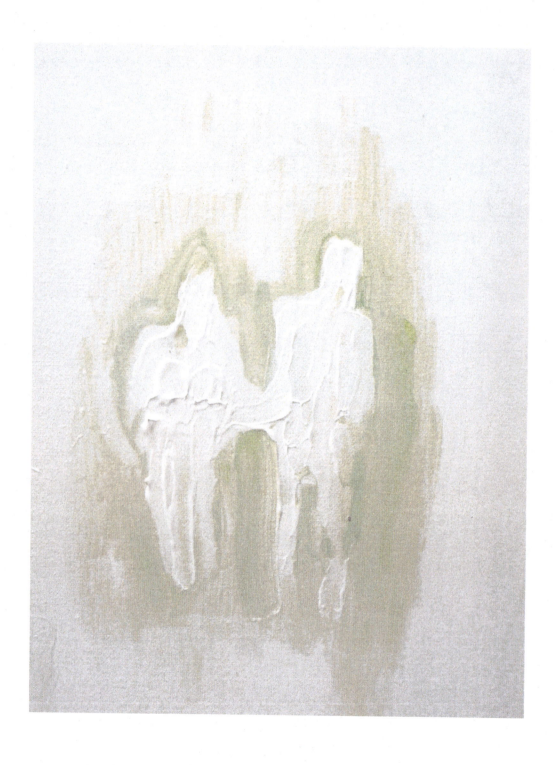

To this day I don't know why I said

> BRENT *(screaming)*
> IT IS FINISHED. IT IS FINISHED!

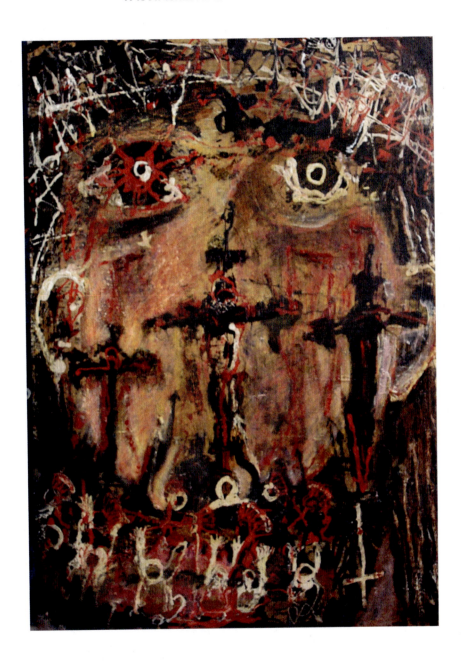

Painted for Artist week at church.
Theme: The last 7 words of Christ.
Bloody Sunday

EXT. JAIL ---------DAY

Brent twists his wrists. The handcuffs are tight, and the policemen walk him out the entrance of the building. The handcuffs are tearing his wrists.
[There is the sound of another helicopter.]

>BRENT (V.O.)
>Shit! We're getting married in jail, AND I am on trial for going through a window... all for my love of E! I am on trial for LOVE. Love for *E* versus the State of Georgia. Well, it's not going to just the local court. I will have to take it to the State Supreme Court. How do I get it there? I MUST emphasize my position for love.

The police back him up against a huge window while handcuffed. Brent hears a helicopter, and sees the landing pad on the roof of the police building. In a flash, Brent slams his foot through the huge, thick, glass window next to the Courthouse door.

>POLICEMAN # 1
>Shit! Ahhh, man. What'd you do that for?

Brent pauses for a short time.

>BRENT
>It's obvious.

>POLICEMAN # 1
>WHAT is obvious?

>BRENT
>You know, I'm emphasizing my position on LOVE versus the State.

>POLICEMAN # 1 (to policeman # 2)
>You hearin' this?

>POLICEMAN # 2
>Dude's nuts, man! And how we going to explain this one!?

>BRENT
>Nuts? I'm just trying to get to a higher court.

> POLICEMAN #2
> Would you shut up!
>
> POLICEMAN # 1
> Son, can you remember what drugs you took and about how long ago? I'd certainly like to know. It could help us better understand.
>
> BRENT (feeling angry for the first time)
> I don't do drugs.

INT. JAIL CHECK-IN ---------DAY

The same two policemen lead him back inside to the check-in area. He sits in a chair. One policeman stands on his left, one on his right. Brent glances at his very dirty and slightly bloody feet. There are shards of glass in his and also. An African American lady slowly kneels down at Brent's feet and removes his sandals. He unsuccessfully fights tears as she washes his feet with a bucket of water and antiseptic. They fingerprint him and take his photo.

INT. JAIL PHONE ---------DAY

> BRENT (in a normal tone of voice)
> Do I get a phone call?

Brent holds a phone to his ear while cuffed.
[Sound of phone RINGING.]

> E. (O.S.)
> Hello?
>
> BRENT
> Hey E. It's Brent. You are not going to believe this. I'm in jail. Will you still marry me?
>
> E. (O.S.)
> Brent?
>
> BRENT
> Yes.

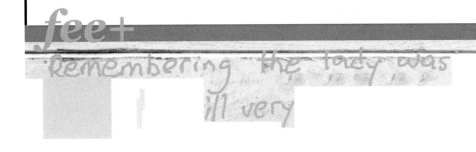

feet
Remembering the lady was ill very

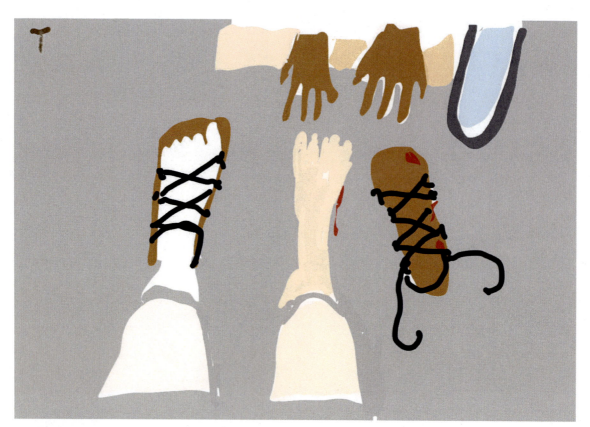

TEARS

r AIN'NG

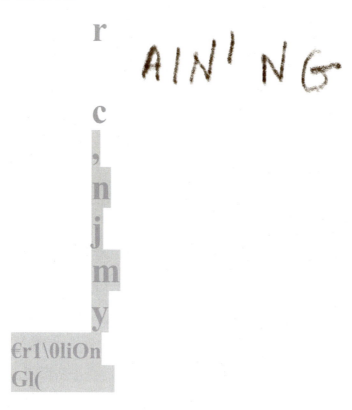

> E. *(0.5.)*
> What are you doing in jail?

> BRENT
> I followed the clues for the wedding.

> E. *(O S.)*
> Brent! You are not in jail, and you didn't just ask me to marry you? This is a joke, right?

> BRENT
> No. Tt is very real. Ts our marriage actually going to be at the jail?

> E. *(0.5.)*
> What are you talking about?

A hand removes the phone from Brent's ear.

> BRENT *(shouting)*
> They are making me get off the phone. I'll stay in contact with you!
> I love you!

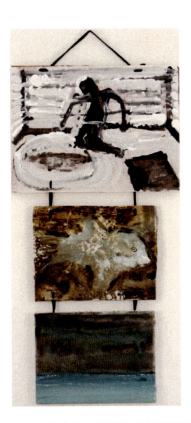

There is a fish within the stormy tears.

INT. TINY CELL----------DAY

Brent holds jail clothes. He has to totally strip, and is now barefoot. He glances at the single, small, smoky window in the cell. His "new" sandals are actually well used.

> BRENT (V.O.)
> A little privacy would be nice.

He reluctantly starts to change. The uniform is solid dark, midnight, policeman blue. The pants fit loosely, but the shirt is very tight. Its shoulders are way up and don't hang down normally. On the shirt, in white, is written "DEKALB COUNTY" and underneath that, "JAIL." Under the word JAIL, is an inch circular, wide dot. He has no underwear. Someone opens a slit in the door and slides a tray of food inside. He takes a tiny bite.

> BRENT (VO.)
> Basic, but this will have to tide me over until the wedding.

He looks up at the grill covering the air-conditioning vent. There is a small piece of paper folded up. It is part of a torn letter.

> BRENT (V.O.)
> This is similar to finding the list of songs in the drainpipe.

He smiles and puts the paper in his pocket. He is unable to concentrate on the small writing.

> BRENT (VO.)
> No one but E would send me notes in jail.

He finishes eating. Someone with a cart passes the outside of the cell. A small piece of paper is stuck under the door. It has letters and symbols, a possible incomplete key to Morse Code.

Brent hears CHILDREN LAUGHING behind the window.

> CHILDREN'S VOICES
> Brent. Brent. Tell us your story, your love for E.

> BRENT (VO.)
> They cannot hear me in here. They are going to bring children into the room opposite this window? I am going to have to break this window so they can hear me on the other side.

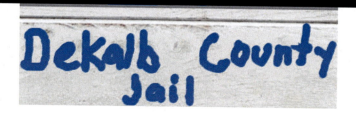

He grabs his food tray and smashes it against the previously cracked window. The window will not break, nor will the tray.

> UNKNOWN VOICE *(in Brent's mind)*
> Are you going to fight for your love?

He smashes the tray harder. The window will not crack any further. It is soon a war, and he loses himself in the fight. He feels the walls of the cell shake. The jail is moving. Someone passes outside the door and says, "God, you are making noise on the other side of the complex." Brent thinks he has broken his hand. He kicks the window with his bare foot, but to no avail. Tears fall. The children's cheers fade. He gives up all hope of ever working with kids. He falls against the window, breathing heavily, and slides down the wall until he's lying on the floor. He feels trapped, and stares at the jail's impenetrable window. His hands are wrapped around the round stool bolted to floor, as if grasping a steering wheel.

INT. CAR ----- LATE NIGHT-------------FLASHBACK

Brent has just been in a near fatal traffic accident with his college friend, and is trapped. Brent is sitting in shock, staring out the car's front window from the driver's side. The window is dark, cracked, and crunched like a horrible fortune cookie. Like tears, the rain is slowly dripping down the outside of the glass. He hears voices of people asking if he is okay. He can't comprehend them. There is a vague memory of looking at a house through the window. Nobody is home at that late hour. The house is dark.

INT. TINY CELL ----------DAY

His eyes fixate on the wall and suddenly he quiets. He slides his fingertips across the wall and down the floor.

> BRENT (VO.)
> You're watching me, aren't you? Who are you? You've censored the walls and the floor. You can feel the heat of my touch.

He writes, "I love you E," on the floor with his finger.

> BRENT (VO.)
> You know exactly what I'm writing, don't you?

He writes, "Evil can't win," with his finger.

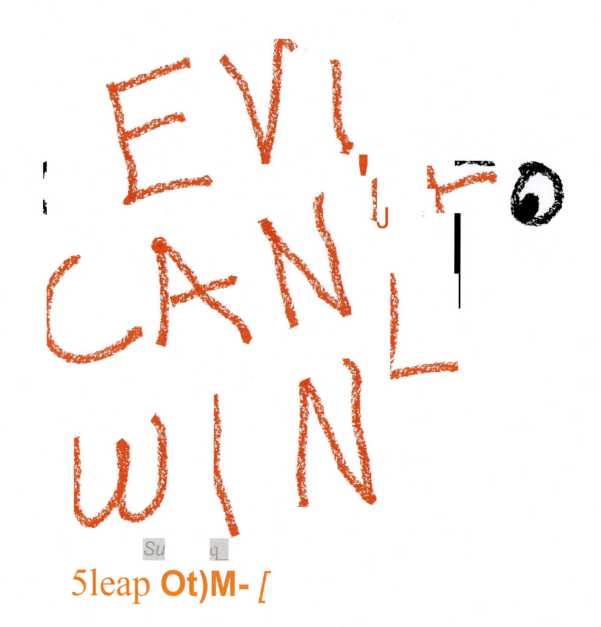

[KEYS JINGLE as footsteps pass by his cell.]

>   *BRENT (V.O (smiling)*
>   My friend, I will call you Saint Peter the sheriff. Why do you have so many keys?

INT. TINY CELL ----- DAY———"FANTASYSEQUENCE"

Brent sees the cell wall as a canvas. He decides to go for an imaginary walk. His hand paints a house in vibran t colors.

STREET
Brent sees a magnolia tree.

TTNYCELL
A hand paints a magnolia tree.

STREET
Brent looks left just in time to see a hand peeling an orange. He looks up at the face, but the body has already walked past him. All he can see is her back.

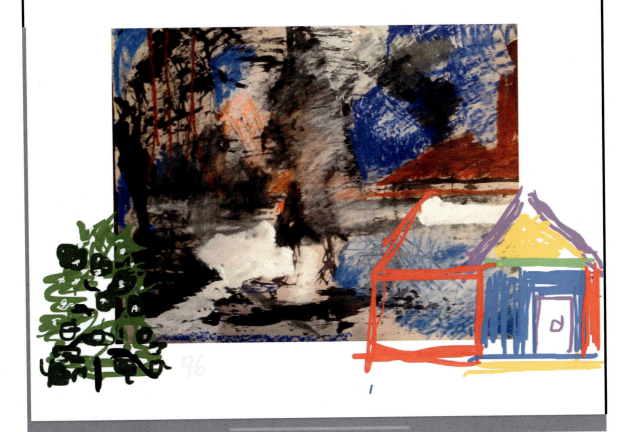

"Walk

TTNYCELL

A hand paints an orange.

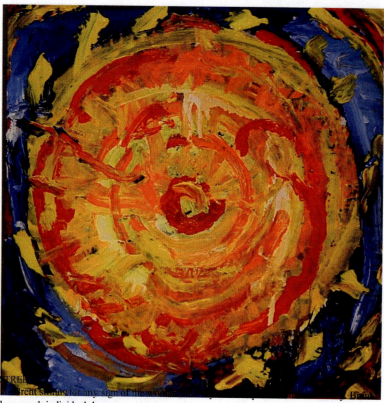

hears each individual drop.

TINY CELL

The drops continue to plop, as the hand paints them on the wall and floor. He notices the temperate differences on the individual walls. The air currents from the vent seem like swirls in a Van Gogh painting.

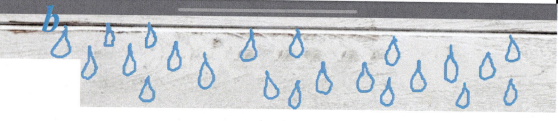

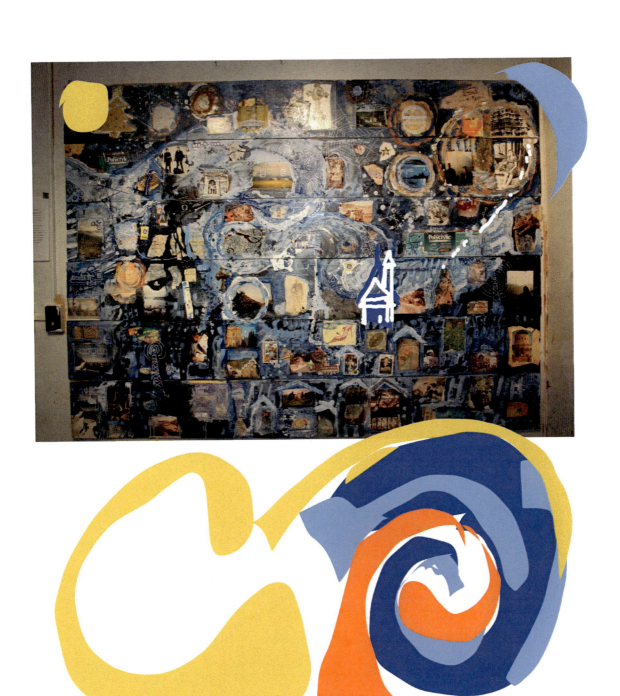

~~INT. TINY CELL ----- DAY/NIGHT UNKNOWN --------END "FANTASY SEQUENCE"~~

Over the house, tree, orange, and wall of rain, Brent draws a purple "E" with his finger. Brent steps back, admires his handiwork. We see nothing on the wall. Brent knocks on his cell door.

          BRENT
          I have to pee.

No response. He writes, "I have to pee," in red paint. No response.

          BRENT (VO.)
          Y'all going to let me out to pee, or you gonna sit there and make me suffer?

Again, he writes in red on the wall, "I have to pee." Again, nothing. Much time goes by as he continues knocking.

          BRENT (VO.)
          This is not fair.

He eyes a milk carton on the floor. LATER

The carton sits on top of the tray in a corner, full.
[A door SHUTTING and LOCKING is heard. In another FLASH, a PISTOL is FIRING. *! possibly at a firing range}* In another FLASH, there is a HAMMER POUNDING a nail into a hand.]

          BRENT (VO.)
          Lord, what am I doing here? Noises here seem evil.

Brent cowers in a corner. He draws a symbol for the noises on the floor. The air conditioning kicks on, making him jolt.

          BRENT (VO.)
          Fresh air; my good friend.

Brent draws what he imagines is the air-conditioning piping system. Positive emotions of having cool air soon fade. He starts shivering uncontrollably. He draws snowflakes on the wall, huddles up in a corner, and puts his ear to the floor.

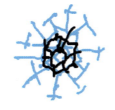
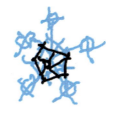
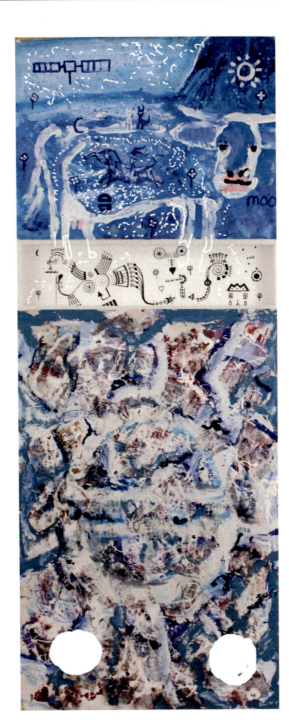

(This painting burned up in a fire on Thanksgiving around '16. I lost ≈100 works.)

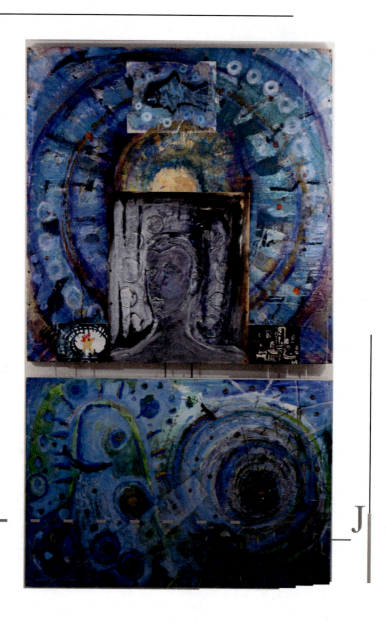

100:-

J

"Cold"

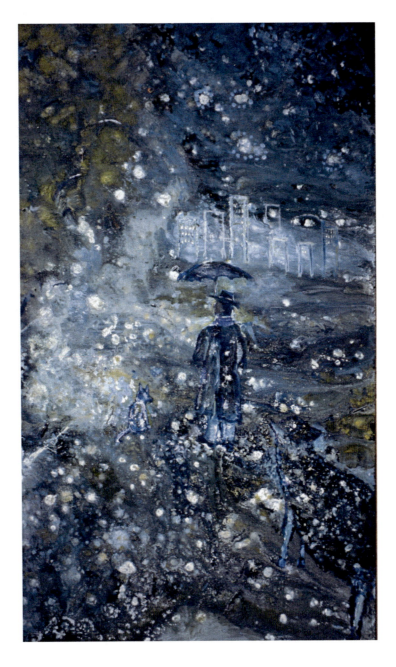

"Leading through the snow"

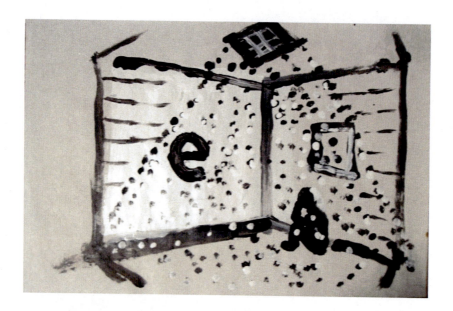

SOUNDS bombard Brent : doors closing, locks clicking, footsteps slappin g, carts rolling, keys jin g ling. While shivering, Brent dra ws a symb ol on the floor for each so und . The sound s repeat fas te r.

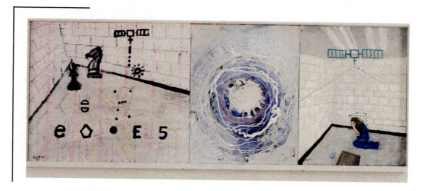

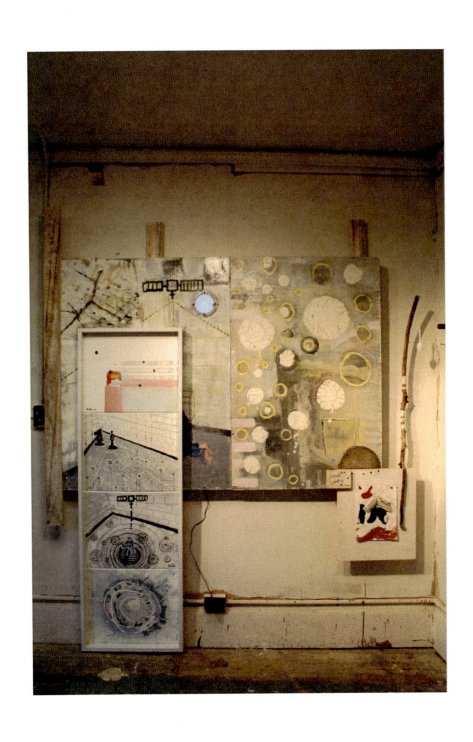

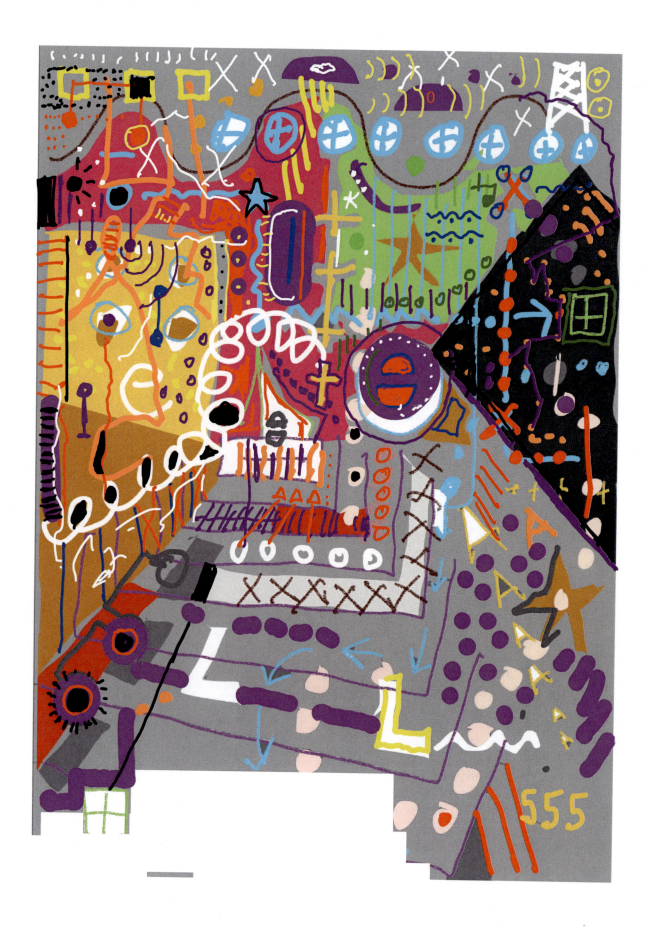

> BRENT (V.O.)
> There are unique codes for different people.

Brent's mind is dancing with, what he perceives as, 50 distinct soun ds. He stops dra wing with his finger; only his ear moves, eve r so slightl y.

> BRENT (VO.)
> My ear is my paintbrush. I use it to dance around the sounds, organizing them, creating art.

A bird chi rps very faintly. Brent assu mes it to be bl ue. Brent takes solace in the friendly bird, and d raws a mu s ical note. He hears a different chi rp slow l y growi ng lou der. ft is d efinit ely a Cardinal. The Cardinal noise soon mixes with silent, sexual, energy waves.

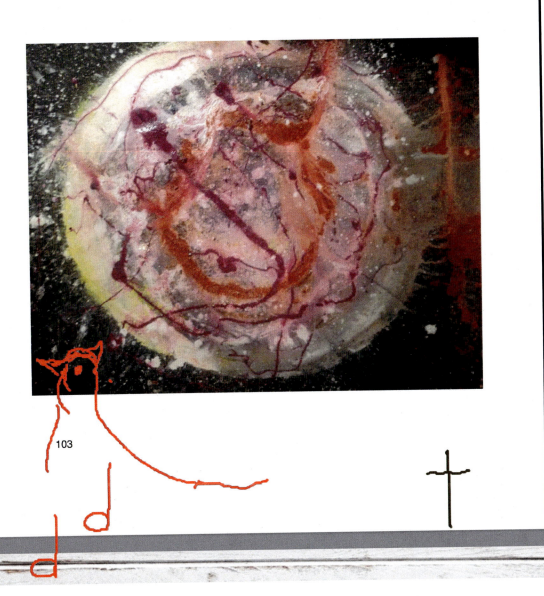

Teroness' c,
ed'
tJri.-ilflrs;-+,
@.*f*:*fr!* '"!:]4

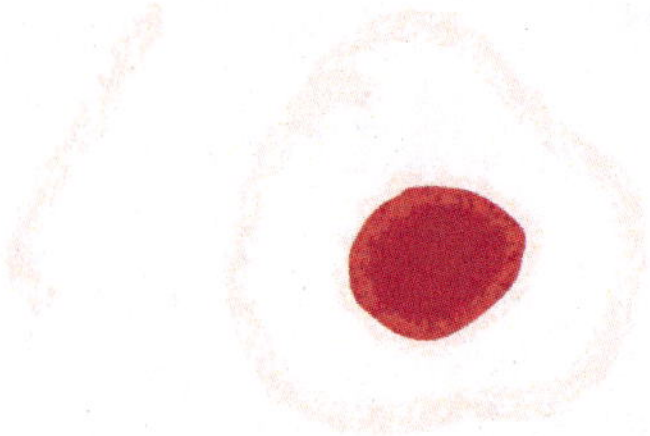

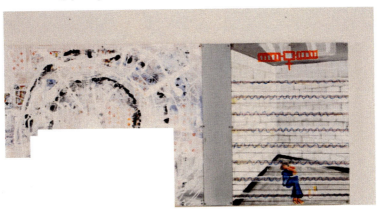

BRENT (V.O.)
Cardinal, is your noise made by a man? Most seductive, most intelligent, most evil of all the noises. Where are you locked up? You sound far away. Is it possible to communicate amongst cells?

Brent, confused, senses a growing evil within the sound. Sexual intensity and vibrations continually fill the cell. The Cardinal chirps again, and Brent is about to explode.

BRENT (V.O.)
What is that, a mating call? Are you calling me? I'm not available. Twill wait for an eventual time with E. You have no business in my space. Feel my heart beat faster and more beautiful than your song.

Brent's heart is pounding loud and fast. Brent's outer appearance is not moving at all. He is caught in a state of suspension, and feels in command of his heartbeat. It finally slows as he wards off the sexual waves of energy. The pace of rhythm slows to a tremendous calm, and for what is an unknown time, Brent feels okay within his white cell, as if some monster had just been avoided. He feels shielded, as consciousness between each heart beat seems like 5 seconds.

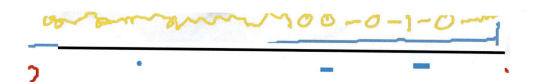

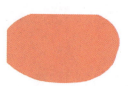

M m m m Madness?

BRENT (VO.)
My heart is my paintbrush. And I can paint like the wind.

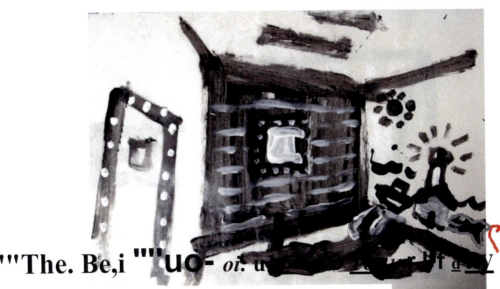

'''The. Be,i ""uO- *oi: u*

THE BEST video of U2's Bad you'll watch TODAY *today*

INT. "GREENHOUSE" ----- DAY ----4 Li sHBAsB):to *where Brent lived a year before the patron sponsored restaurant series)*

Brent's friend, Mike, stops by and wakes Brent from deep slumber. He is on the top bunk and is dazed, not getting up right away. He is caught between dreams and reality. Brent just stares out the window. Mike just looks at Brent and then exits up to the living room. An unknown time later, Brent gets up and goes to the living room, still dazed. He finds his roommates, plus Mike, engrossed in the latest episode of *Star Trek: the Next Generation*. The episode is titled, *Frame of Mind*.

ROOMMATE #1
Lieutenant Riker is imprisoned within his own brain!

Brent looks towards a part eaten sandwich on the table.

b. Flq rhb'1c: k to
Cc.rleDrern

This ntni, comes from notes and a
Flash-back to Cafe Diem

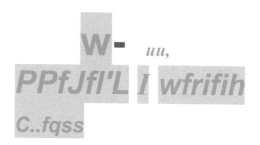 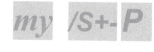

"Greenhouse"

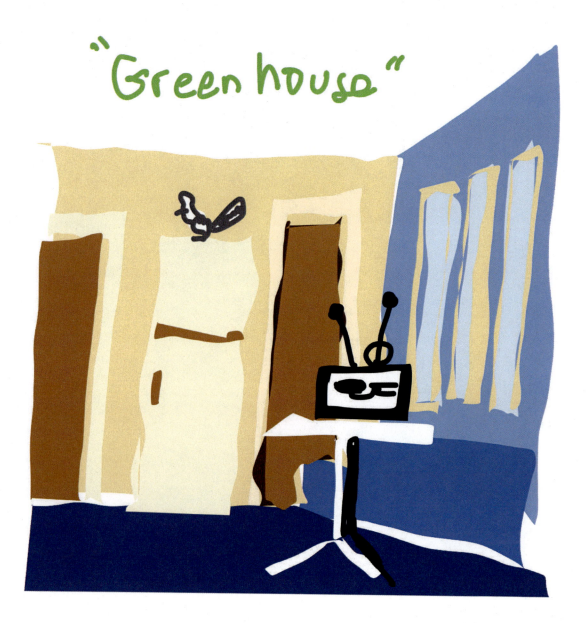

Bonnie the tame squirrel is on the fridge. She would come down the tree outside, climb on the roof, to our shoulder and eat cheese.

> BRENT
> Isn't he "Second in Command" aboard the *Enterprise?*

> ROOMMATE#2
> Not at the current moment. Psychological levels within his own consciousness are being controlled by a mind alternating machine in the hands of a mad poli tician.

> ROOMMATE#3
> We are having a difficult time distinguishing Riker's conscious
>
> realities.

"Riker, just calm down!"

> BRENT *(whispering to Mike)*
> Is it Riker, or my roommates, being controlled by a machine?

> RIKER *(from the TV screams)*
> What's REEEAL!?

Brent pretends to be recouping from sleep. During the next commercial, he echoes the scream softly. He shakes his head and badgers Mike.

> BRENT *(seriously, but jokingly)*
> "What is real?"

Nobody answers except for the TV commercial man selling the new Q Infinity car.

> Q INFINITY MAN
> "... Q Infinity"

Brent stares directly at the eyes of his roommates.

> BRENT *(howling)*
> What is real? WHAT IS REEEEAL?

Mik etakes notice, and slowly turns towards Brent with weird, strange, and subtle facial

expressions. Brent's eyes widen and his eyebrows furl, making for a double take. Mike has surprised him. Brent has been phased and transported into a show that he actually does like.

> Okay, Mike. You got me. I'm now warped into the show. Quickly catch me up with more details.

Brent is hooked into a machine until Riker is not. The show is soon over.

> BRENT
> Hey Mike, I am hungry, and I have a "written" paper due for Painting I. I have to critique a gallery.

> MTKE
> T didn't wake you up just to watch *Star Trek*. Want to go to Cafe Diem?

> BRENT
> I can't afford to get into the High Museum. There are some paintings at Cafe Diem, aren't there?

> MIKE
> And some painted tables too. I'll buy ya beer, if you want.

> BRENT
> I'm in! I will call *E* and see if she wants to go.

Mike smirks.

> BRENT
> Why not? You have been asking about her, and she has been asking about you.

> MIKE
> Calling *E* is YOUR idea.

> BRENT
> Yeah, you bet! Besides, I've got this PAPER to write. Y'all can do most of the talking. It's what you want, isn't it?

INT. CAFE DIEM ---------EVENING

Cafe Diem is in Virginia Highlands. It has a sidewalk European flair. All the inside, round tables are painted differently.

108

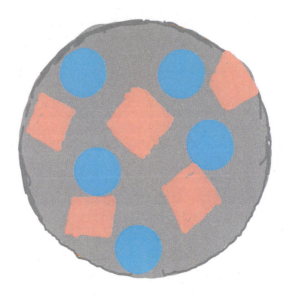

> MTKE
> Maybe my favorite table will be open.

Mike grins and points.

> BRENT
> That's your table?

Mike steers Brent and *E* to the table. It is round, nuovo, modern pastel pink and blue dots, on a grey background.

> MTKE
> What's wrong with it?

> BRENT
> Nothing. Kitsch has its place. Think it matches the adobe tiled floor?

> E.
> I LIKE this table. GOOD choice, Mike.

E looks at Mike intently, and Mike looks at Brent with a sarcastic smile.

E is still looking at Mike.

> E.
> Have you ever eaten here? What do you recommend to eat?

Brent makes a goofy face as he looks at Mike.

> MIKE
> The chicken salad croissant and grapes are pretty good.

Waiter in vogue arrives with glasses of water.

> WAITER
> Can I start you with something else to drink? Coffee? Wine?

> E.
> What wine would you recommend with the chicken salad croissants?

> WATTER
> *(unknown name of wine);* it's French.

> MIKE
> I'd like a Stella Artois.

> BRENT
> Hmmmmm? I need a few more minutes.

Mike and *E* start talking about the weekly Bible study they all are a part of.

> E.
> Mike, I've got some concerns about the teachings regarding women and the church.

Brent slowly scans the room with a quick look at the art hanging from the walls. Brent looks at £.

> BRENT
> Haven't you and I already talked about this.

E just stares at Brent.

Brent smiles and winks at *E*.

E, without any hesitation or response, turns back to Mike.

> E.
> Do you think women can have a pastoral or an organizational leadership role within the church, i.e. Perimeter Ministries International or PCA?

Waiter returns with drinks.

> BRENT
> I'll take the roast beef and banana slices and a bottled Coca-Cola. Oh, if you have an extra pen and napkins, I would appreciate it as well.

> WATTER *(smiles)*
> Sure!

E stills the conversation as pen and paper napkins are quietly slipped in front of Brent. She swirls her wine.

> *E.*
> This will be really good with dinner.

Brent is eager to look at the art; he doesn't want to start a new conversation about wine.

> *BRENT*
> Y'all, is it okay if I check out of the conversation for awhile? Besides, T don't know much about wine. T need to take some notes about the art on the walls here. T have a WRTTIEN paper for Painting I?! It's already way overdue. It's suppose to be from a gallery visit, but here will have to do.

E seems a little disappointed as her and Mike's food arrives.

> *E. and MIKE*
> No problem.

> *BRENT*
> Sweet!

> *E.*
> Mike, I think PCA has got it wrong.

Brent stares at the art around the room. He slowly and disappointedly analyzes all the paintings in the room. Taking notes on the napkins as he goes, he looks at the hues, textures, tinctures, opacities, and intensities.

> *BRENT (VO.)*
> These painting vocab words are missing the point.

[There is a guitarist] The scent of coffee reminds him of Bordeaux. The fashions dancing around are not typical for Atlanta . Bones take on the beat of the strum of the guitar .
There is a fan and a wonderful kitsch painting of a big coffee cup, behind the cash register. Brent is mesmeri zed by the whirling fan, and the sounds of the cash register begin to drown out peripheral perception. Brent retreats into the recesses of his mind. *E* and Mike have been talking about a new topic, but Brent doesn 't knowwhat.

> *BRENT (interrupting excitedly)*
> Look at THAT painting!

BRENT points to the large window. On the other side of the glass is a porch, a tree, and people sitting. [The porch is dark with a light shining up into the tree.]

> E. *(excited)*
> What are you talking about?

> BRENT
> Come on! Look at that painting... the WINDOW! It's alive. It's REAL, dammit! Conversations are only visual and cannot be heard. They hint at stories that have no end ... what a strange mark on his arm?

> E. *(Smiles)*
> I follow! I don't care for that tattoo.

> BRENT
> Man look at THAAAAAAT HAAAT! Just where do you think she got it?

> E.
> No telling around here. It's cool!

> BRENT
> Remember that mushroom hat you were wearing when I first met you "again" at my parent's house? It was way cooler.

> MIKE *(jokingly confused)*
> Wait, whose hat has what? And whose hat is whose... on whom?

> BRENT
> The man... his cigarette... is it really burning? The beer in the tall, erect glass... it's half full, while the other half is expressed in the color of his face.

On the other side of the window, a tall, bodacious woman is on the lap of another man whose back is turned. He turns and shows his homely face.

> BRENT
> She is resting there. Why him? He must have something more than that simple brown coat.

[From below, a ground light illumines the tree, casting people's shadows into the top of the tree.]

> E.
> Murmurs of love. Maybe that's the topic of conversation.

E smiles and takes a sip of her remaining wine.

> BRENT (pointing at window)
> E, what's that painting by Renoir of everyone outside in a scene kind of similar to that, hats and all?

> E.
> Oh, you must be talking about *The Luncheon on the Boating Parh;*. I do believe that was 18... 81.

> BRENT
> Holy shit! That's it. How do you remember that stuff?

> E.
> I'm smart, remember!

> BRENT *(smiling)*
> You are not even a Fine Arts Major. You must have had Art History.

E smiles at Brent.

Brent starts to fidget a little and looks back at the menu to check the price of another bottled Coca-Cola.

> BRENT (looking at Mike)
> Maybe I'll get a BEER. **T** s till have **to** look at more of the art on the walls. My paper has to be soooo lo ng.

E and Mike both agree they have time. Mike doesn't remember about buying the beer for Brent. Brent soon forgets too, as he sees the back of the menu. Brent's eyes go wide.

> BRENT
> Oh my God! *The Lun cheon on the Boating Party* is on the back of the menu! *Eeeeeee?*

> E.
> What?

> BRENT
> Did you see that picture on the menu a minute ago?

> E.
> NO! Did you?

> BRENT
> I don't know! This is plain luck, Jungian *syn chronicity,* or God revealed.

> E.
> Let's go with synchronicity. Pretty amazing.

E winks at Brent. Brent doesn't know how to handle the wink.

> BRENT
> We will never know.

Brent looks again at the menu. The beer and the bottled Coke cost more than he really wants to spend. Mike is finishing the last of his grapes.

> MIKE
> We gotta come back here again.

E notices Brent is now looking at the art again and taking notes; she prolongs conversation.

> E.
> Agreed! Mike, what do you think?...

Looking again at the art on the walls, Brent writes on the napkins some final words: "Left

over hippie art, the kind that hinted at old artistic movements without the

creative struggle for something new. Surrealisms, 'Whateverisms,' all lacking the wrestle with the demon and the dialogue with the priest. I better stop the negativity, cause I do the same."

> BRENT
> That's the only painting here not for sale.

He points to the big coffee cup painting behind the register.

> E.
> I think the owner likes that one. You know, it has a sister painting over there. I like it:8 rose on the piano.
>
> BRENT
> Have y'all heard of Richard Roarty and his theory on *dialogue?* Does it concern visual language also?

Mike and E just stare at Brent.

> BRENT *(smiling at E)*
> Come on E, you ARE smart. [Pause] E

looks directly at Brent.

> E.
> Brent, is this a gallery, or a CAFE?
>
> BRENT
> This table and window is a reality I'm going to have to return to one day.
>
> MIKE
> So, how do you like the TABLE?
>
> E. *(looking at Brent seriously, then smiling at Mike)*
> Mike, thank you for the CONVERSATION. *(Subtly)* And the table was a really good choice; we will have to come back again.

Brent just stares out the window.

> BRENT
> You know, in class, I just did a painting in encaustic of my garage door window from childhood.
>
> E
> At GA State, or at GA TECH? I know you have been cross enrolling?

7. Sounds S-mr+ analthe Orcan-'e. *C:rlow*

Sounds Start + the Orange Glow

        BRENT
        GA State, the concrete campus. It is my first painting class.

        E.
        You know, I teach English on Tues. and Thurs. I'm not far from the Art Department. Maybe I can stop by some time.

        BRENT
        I'd like that. Professor Holden is really cool; he also runs a grist mill once a month up in north GA somewhere.

Mike's interest is perked.

        MIKE
        That sounds like a good day trip for a weekend.

£ smiles.

        £. (seriously)
        Yeah, we should definitely go sometime. But I am going to have to go for now, got PAPERS to grade.

INT. SMALL JAIL CELL   **<DAY/NIGHT UNKNOWN)**

[Suddenly, a SLAM, followed by SILENCE, then a strange TONE on the periphery of normal hearing is heard. The tone turns into very fast, interrupting beeps. Electricity is heard, and fluorescent lights are barely vibrating .] Bren t's body shivers violently. He is freezing. The frequency of lighting makes Brent squint.

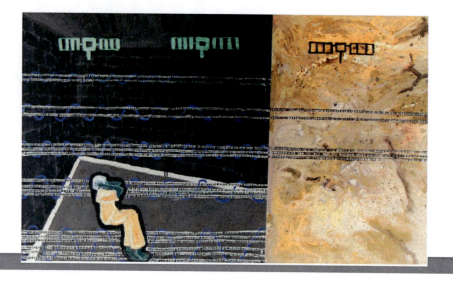

> BRENT (V.O.)
> Oh my God! Please, some quiet.

Brent slides over to the other corner, covers his ears, and begins to rock, as waves of energy shudder through him.

> BRENT
> Where's the source? Leave ME alone.

> BRENT (V.O.)
> God, the energy... it's all sexual... they're raping me! They want me to participate!

> BRENT
> I WON'T DO IT!

He smashes a packet of mayonnaise on the door. He then covers his ears with his hands and slides to a different corner. The waves soften.

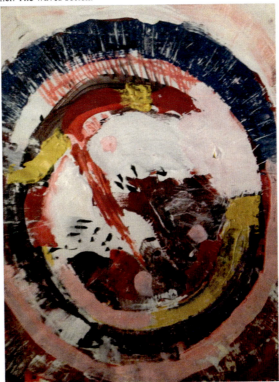

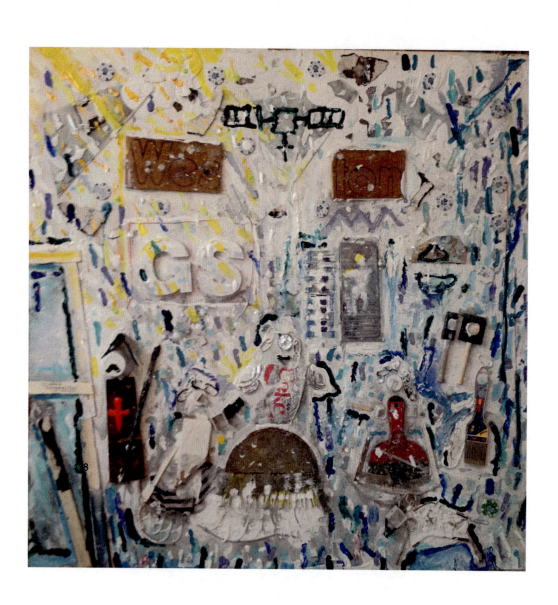

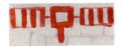

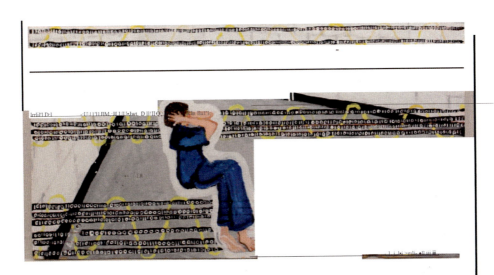

Andy your sermons are the opposite of this painting.

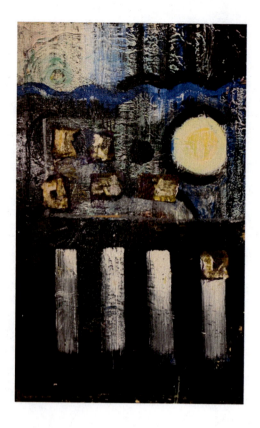

                    BRENT (VO.)
                    Hope.

The waves settle. Brent is stunned, and looks around the cell. He removes his hands from his ears slowly. All remains silent. He breathes deep.

                    BRENT
                    Thank you, God!

[SCRATCHING NOISES comes from the wall.]

                    BRENT (VO.)
                    Now, that sounds like *E*. The sounds seem to match her
                    personality. The scratching sound s like what her pen marks

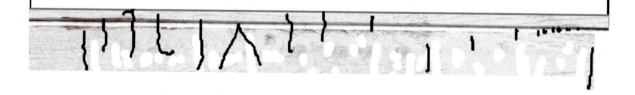

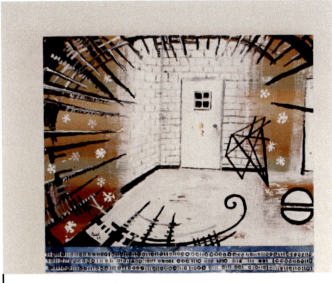
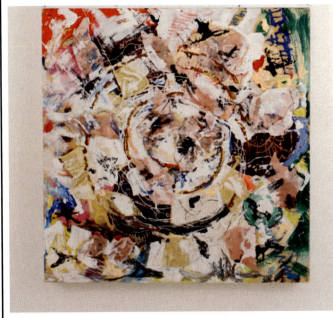

wou ld make on paper... a soft touch. In the upper classes at GA Sta
te, weren't they studying sounds made in the process of drawing?

He slams his ear against the wall.

> BRENT
> E? Have they got you locked up, too?

[More scratching.]

> BRENT (V O.)
> Talk to her. How can I talk to her?

He scra tches on the wall, but can not interpret the responsive, new sound.

> BRENT (V.0.)
> Brent, that doesn't mean anything.

He writes, "I love you," on the wall with his finger. No response. He draws a line for the word "I", two curved lines for a heart, and a curvy "U".

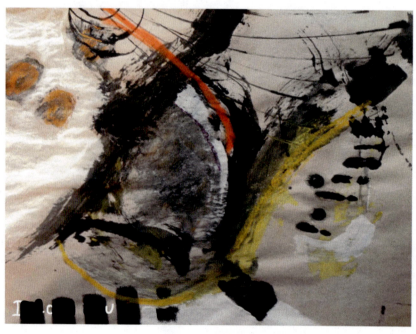

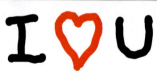

> BRENT
> E, what do you want me to do? How can we understand each other?

[More scratching.] He writes, "Talk to me E," on the wall.

> BRENT (VO.)
> Romeo and Juliet in jail.

[Keys jingle] He smiles. GUARD opens the door. Brent smiles.

> GUARD A
> Let's go.

Brent obeys.

INT. COMMON CELL E1A ---------DAY

The door opens into a large, drab, yellow / orang"is h" room filled with dirty bw1k-beds, heavy smoke, and approximately twenty inmates. Orange, fluorescent bulbs seem to make the room vibrate. A Guard gives Brent a roll of toilet paper, a towel, and sheets, then escorts him inside. Brent walks to an empty bed in the back on the right. Ashes lay on the W1inv iting, bare mattress.

His eyes are drawn immediately to the window of the door into the common room.

> BRENT (VO.)
> That window looks breakable. That doesn't make sense!

The Atlanta Braves are playing on the TV, but the reception cuts in and out. Brent scans the cell studying his new ROOMMATES, a mangy gang of guys. He notices right away a guy with a small radio tied to his headband that covers his right ear. There is no antenna on RADIOMAN'S radio. ROOMMATES are trading "roll-ups" for "moonpies."

Brent feels a beam of light pour down on him from above. It shoots in a straight line down over his head and through his body. It seems to sink into the depths of the floor, taking him with it. He lifts his face up to feel the warmth, but feels like he is in a mental elevator descending into a dark pool of waves. He is sinking into a web.

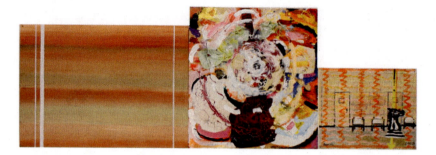

JOE, a burly guy in the bed next to Brent, doesn't see the light; the light disappears. Brent brushes the ashes off his bed as best he can, makes it, and crawls in. Brent cannot sleep, as Joe is in bed a few feet away, playing with his own pecker. Brent tries to understand the personality types of the people in the big room. The only person he trusts after a cursory look, is the guy that never moves, except to eat.

LATER

Brent is awakened by an unintelligible mix of profanity and judgment day Bible verses streaming from the mouth of one of his neighbors. This neighbor is locked in an adjoining cell off the main room. The screaming goes on and off for hours. Brent has never heard words in Eng lish screamed unconnectedly with so much force or for so
lo ng.

> BRENT (VO.)
> God, I need some sleep. These guys are really crazy.

Another neighbor in a locked room, stops up his commode. Water, wit h a turd, flows out from under the door next to Brent's bed. Brent gets up and wanders arow1d the communal cell. He looks at the doors into the other adjoining individual cells. One door opens with "Radioman." He is in charge of the "store."

One door window is surrounded by severa l men looking in. Brent looks over their shoulders, and he sees a man wearing a white toga made from bed sheets; his body is covered in sores. The man is sitting on a bed doing obscene acts. Fairy like drawings, literally drawn on the walls, cover the dingy, low light, orange room that has no windows. Brent sits down to eat at a table bolted to the floor. There are two identical

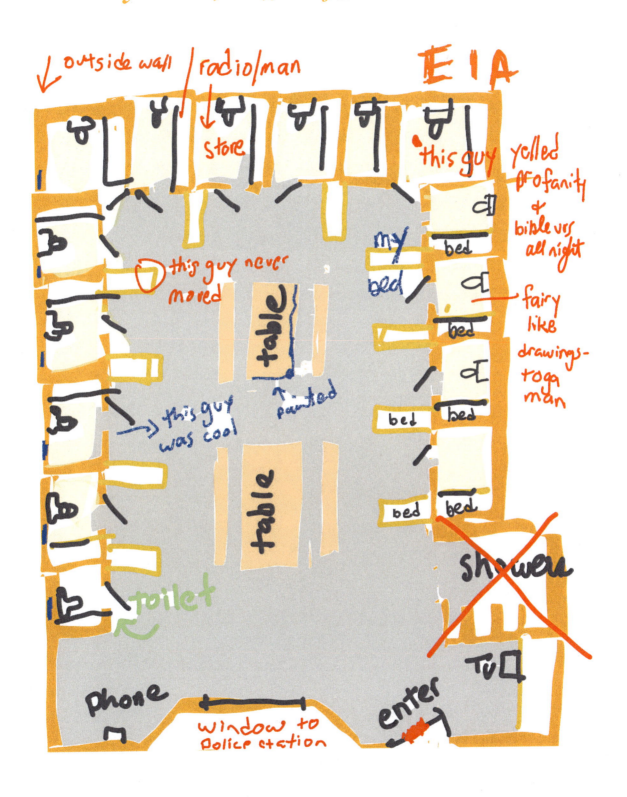

g. The T'-'ble. *Tvrnt*

tables. One is smooth, freshly painted without a scratch. The other has years of scratches and carvings in the paint, revealing past colors of the table. Brent thinks the second a tremendous work of art. He goes to study it. His hand traces some of the marks of names, drawings...

> BRENT (VO.)
> Why fresh paint one table and not the other?

8. The Table Turns

INT. GA. STATE ART DEPARTMENT ----- DAY ------------FLASHBACK

Brent is in the painting studio at GA State. His hand is softly following the lines on an art school table that has years of subconscious painting on it. He is in the process of making his own marks on the table. *E* walks through the doors into the art studio. Her hair is long, and she is carrying a very artistic purse. She is wearing heels and looks like someone walking out of Vogue Magazine. She is wearing lime-green and frosted orange. She smiles at Brent excitedly as she walks toward him. Brent stops and watches her approach.

> E.
> Hey Brent, so sorry I'm a little late.

She does not really care about being late.

> BRENT
> It's no problem. How ya doing?

> E.
> Quite well, thank you. What a nice space! The windows are LARGE, and the lighting is GREAT! What you working on?

> BRENT
> Doing what I do I best. I'm painting.

> E.
> So, you are smearing pigments... right onto a school table?

Brent laughs to himself.

> BRENT
> Actually, I am pouring paint on it and

Brent points to a brush from the side of the table with his woode n paint case. *E* notices the paint box, but doesn't say anything.

>E.
>What's up with the table?

>BRENT
>In Painting I, there are several things I'm working on. Professor Holden sometimes picks up a chair, or a piece of paper or something. Then he looks underneath it without an explanation. T'm pretty sure it has to do with a different way of viewing... asking the CONCEPTUAL questio n, "What is UNDERNEATH?"... meaning look DEEPER. I cannot help but look at my earlier encaustic painting of my child hood window and feel a little remorse. Under the encaustic is just -b ought canvas substratum...

Brent points at the encaustic painting.

>£. *(in terrup ting)*
>The table!?

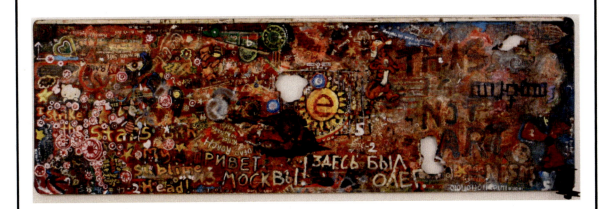

who wrote "this is NotArt" on the table?
&
who wrote in Russian?

BRENT
I was getting there. The TABLE presents a more rich, alive, and historically laden substratum . The assignment was to do a self portrait I have started making marks over these subconscious, and purposeful, paint strokes. Part of ME is engaging the marks that came before me. I also talk with people as they paint on my self-portrait. My argument... part of ME is the dialogue with other people, both verbally and visually.

Brent points to the unintentional, and intentional, marks.

E.
So, you may actually be projecting part yourself onto the table. Is the table you, or PART of you? Are all the projections you? Are YOU just the dialogue?

BRENT
Good questions. I'll have to think on these. Does the painted "on" become just a projection of the "self?" When does the painting stop becoming part of the painter? When the actual painting process is stopped, or is it when the creator, or viewer, is no longer engaged with the art?

E.
It may always live somewhere in the memory of the artist! Or in the memory of the viewer! Or even on a computer screen!

BRENT
I'm getting mixed up now. Wish Carl Jung was here. Anyway, I am inviting other people to paint on the table with me... to dialogue in the process, and see where the life of the painting goes, how it affects me, and how it IS me.

E.
You are raising some interesting questions about the "self."

BRENT
I know. Want to paint?
Without hesitation in her nice teaching clothes.

E.
Pick out some thing blue and green.

> BRENT
> You got it.

> E.
> What kind of paint is this?

> BRENT
> Acrylic, remember I'm allergic to oil.

> E.
> Looks l ike the top is almost finished. Any room underneath?

Brent looks pu zzled.

> BRENT
> I'll turn it over and get you some brushes.

> E.
> Forget the brushes! Squeeze some paint out on a palette.

Brent's eyes widen as he turns the table over.

> BRENT
> Okay?

E proceeds to take her hands and dip them directly into the acrylic paint. She rubs her hands on the underside of the table.

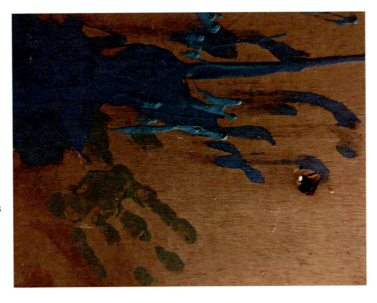

Since '93, every year I have painted on this table, or had someone else do it.

9. Bloody *J-fq"d* at EJA

When she is done, she looks at the paint case.

        E.
Bet they haven't seen a paint case like that in Painting I. Have you named it?

        BRENT
Nope, but it IS one of a kind.

● **<u>INT. ORANGE COMMON CELL E1A ---------DAY</u>**
The architecture gives off noises like a belly of a dragon. Radioman, a muscular African American, joins Brent at the "carved into" table. He blows smoke directly into Brent's face. Brent coughs.

        RADTOMAN
Are you sayin' my breath stinks?

        BRENT
What?

        RADIOMAN
'Cause if you are, I'm saying your breath stinks, and not just your breath, but your whole body smells like you spent the night in a trash compactor.

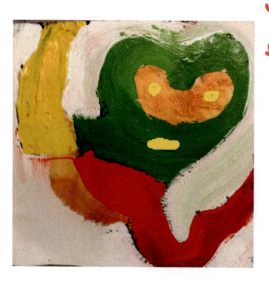

Brent pours a cup of water on Radioman's hand, extinguishing his cigarette. Radioman nails Brent with a right hook that knocks him off the table bench. Brent moans, gets up, and goes to his bed. His roll of toilet paper is gone.

"Who took my roll of toilet paper?"

INMATE walks through the cell picking up food trays. Brent gets up and snags the plastic spoon off his tray. He slides it into his pocket.

          BRENT (V.O.)
          Suppose to rum all utensils back in. This is the first thing I can call MINE in a long time. Ownership, the key to survival in jail?

An inmate tells Brent not to go where everyone "fakes" showers. Brent stays away from that spot his whole time in the common cell.

Meanwhile, Brent plays with the spoon. He uses it to launch little pieces of scrunched up paper. He places crumpled up paper at points where there seems to be an electrical hotspot within the room. The hotspots of the cell are like acupuncture points within the architecture. Someone asks, "What is he doing?"

          NATIVE AMERICAN (with long hair and severe acne, yells) This guy is a genius! He doesn't need our games to entertain; he makes them up. He's a shaman.

          BRENT (V.O.)
          I may be smart, but I know I am no genius, and DEFINITELY no shaman.

That night, when the lights are down and many are asleep, Brent jumps up on the one table that is freshly painted. He takes off his tight, undersized jail shirt. He starts to lower his pants. The custodial inmate walks out of an adjoining cell and asks him what he is doing. Brent is not sure. The custodial man tells him sharply, "Stop!" and to put his shirt back on. Brent goes back to his bed wondering what just happened. Brent cannot

sleep. In the morning, the man that never moves except to eat, is in line for the kool-aid and holds his cup under the spout. He presses the nozzle, totally missing the cup. On purpose, he lets it pour all over the floor. Brent sees someone spit. Because of the close confines, he realizes that in whatever direction one spits, will be in the direction of a particular person.

          BRENT (V.O.)
          If I have to spit, it will be towards my own feet, and I will let it drop. Don't want to look like I'm spitting AT someone.

INT. TV COMMON ROOM EIA   **DAY OR NIGHT?**

Later, Brent looks at the TV.

> BRENT (VO.)
> That guy looks like me.

Brent stands up. The guy on TV stan ds up. Brent scratches his head. The guy on TV scratches his head.

> BRENT (VO.)
> That guy is copying me in a slight delay! That's us up there . People are acting us out on TV. Maybe. Maybe not.

He sits down. The guy on TV sits down.

> BRENT (V O.)
> Only one way to find out. I can't just si t here not knowing if he's copying me.

Brent looks around the room. No one is watching him. He looks at the door window he passed when brought to the common room. The guy on TV looks at a window.

> BRENT (V O.)
> This is too weird .

Brent slinks over to the window. Nobody pays attention to him. He puts his fist through the window on the first try. People in the cell go nuts except for the man who just sits on his bed abso lut ely motionless.

> INMATES (scream ing all at once)
> Fuck! Glass! Blood!

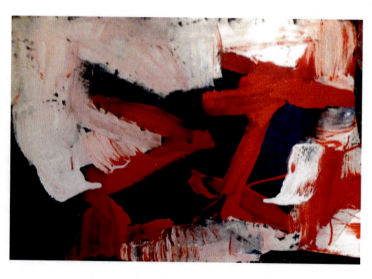

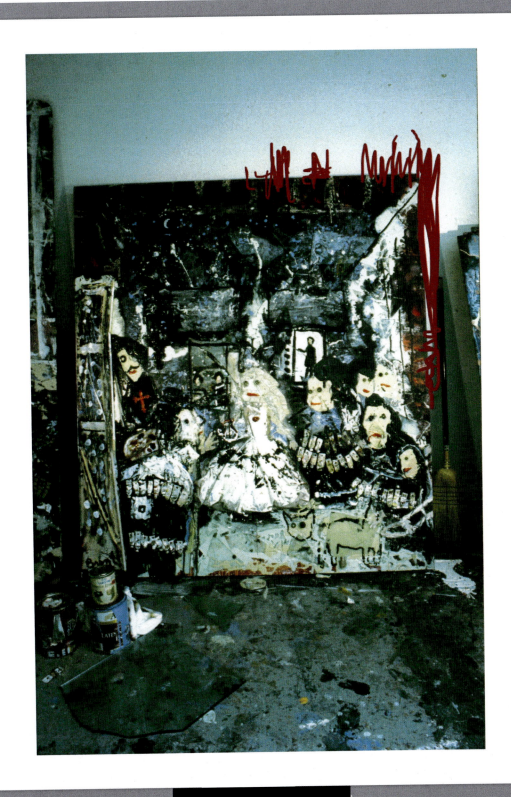

m ₁ ‾ *P*   @(.(ms   *Yi*;,.;

•p   in
              1

all art is the same an attempt to fill empty space
 Samuel Beckett

Before him stood The tree, His Tree, if you could say that of a tree that was alive.

J.R.R. Tolkien, Leaf by Niggle.
us

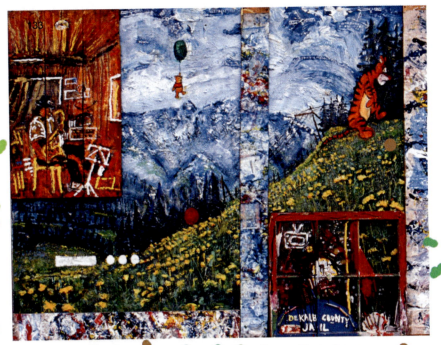
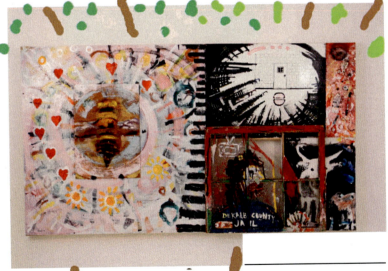

Guards hurry in. Brent's hand pours blood. A Guar d grabs Brent.

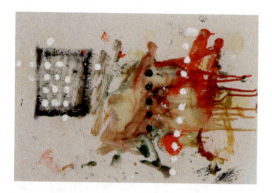

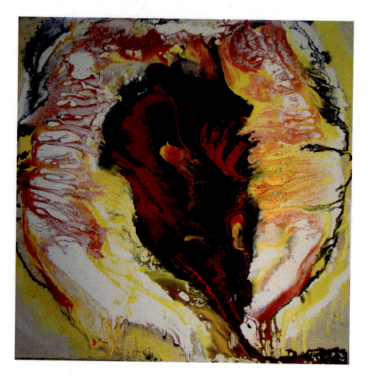

Seeing my hand bleed was freaky.

> GUARD A *(to Guard B)*
>
> Is this the same guy who got the Courthouse window the other day?
>
> BRENT *(interrupting)*
>
> Why the hell do you guy8 have a breakable window in here? Do you have any concept of how 8tupid that i8? Some of the8e guy8 are definite felons and would kill each other with that glass!

Guard A walks Brent out of the room.

> GUARD A
>
> Has it occurred to you that you didn't have to break it?
>
> BRENT
>
> Nope . I had to break it. I had to know if that guy on TV was copying me.
>
> GUARD A
>
> Man, be quiet!

INT. JAIL NURSING STATION---------DAY

Brent's hand is now wrapped in a cloth bandage by a large, overweight, very effemin ate, African American, male nur se. Brent is glad his hand has been cleaned. Blood leaks its way through the top of the bandage. He will have a scar on top of his right hand for life.

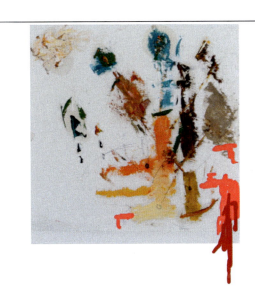

INT. SWISS CHALET: L'ABRI ----- NIGHT --------------FLASHBACK

Inside a door of a Swiss chalet at L'Abri, Brent and a female friend are seriously talking. They are talking about doubts of God and good verses evil. Brent is directly right next to the door. Outside the window, it is rainy and dark over the valley. Lightening is in the background. The chalet is dimly lit. A face of a LONC HAIRED CUY quickly appears pressed up against the window next to Brent. Brent turns toward the window and is spooked badly. His hand crashes through the window towards the face.

> LONG HAIRED MAN (talking through the broken window)
> Brent, it is me, Richard. You okay?

> BRENT
> God, Ri chard, you frig h tened me! Are YOU okay?

Brent look s down at his hand. He is embarrassed that he jumped uncontro llab ly and put his hand th rough the window.

> BRENT
> I think my hand is cut. How about your face?

> RICHARD
> Sorry about that! Didn't mean to scare you that bad.

Richard laughs.

> RICHARD
> I think the glass scratched my nose.

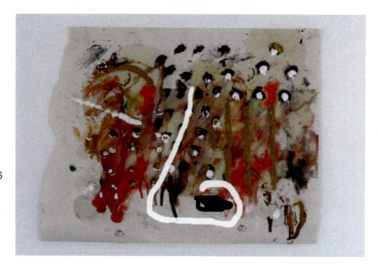

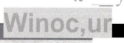

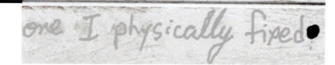

INT. WHITE JAIL CELL (VOICES) -------------NIGHT OR DAY?

10. Mental Sounds + Audible Images of people

Bre n t is ushered into a large cell with white, concrete blocks and Plexi-glass windows. He is

alone. Through the wind ows, Brent can see the lobby with a large security s tation. Brent stud ies the frames of the windows. The braces benea th are upside dow n crosses. He thinks of Pe ter who was crucifie d up side down. He writes continu o us lower case "e"s in cursive on the walls with his hand. They appear in red. They look similar to some of Cy Twombly's late work. The "e"s also look like rolled barbed wire.

> BRENT
> E you are LIFE!

[The ELECTRICAL NOISES a nd ENERGY WAVES retu rn.]

> BRENT (VO.)
> Oh, SHIT, not again.

The in tensified gravity and energy waves become an invisible mass of unbearable wei g ht, a ll res tin g on Brent's should ers. It is too heavy to bare. Brent groans and bend s at the wais t.

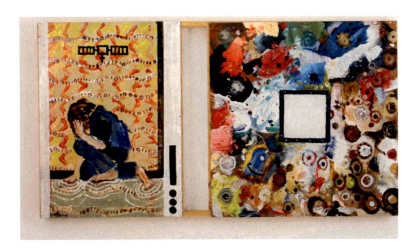

137

                    BRENT (V.O.)
            I feel the weigh t of ten thousand pounds . This ain't good! I'm losing
            control of my lungs!

His knees buckle, and the weight pushes him all the way down to the floor until he's lying smashed flat, on his belly.

GEOMETRIC SYMBOLS flash before his clos ed eyes in rap id successio n. They a ppear as different m il itary in si gnias.

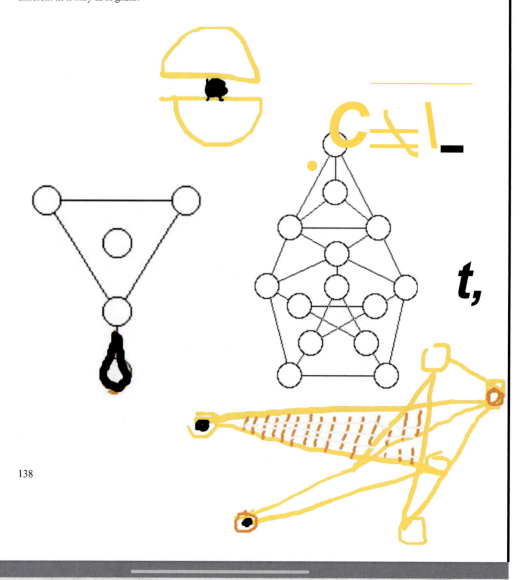

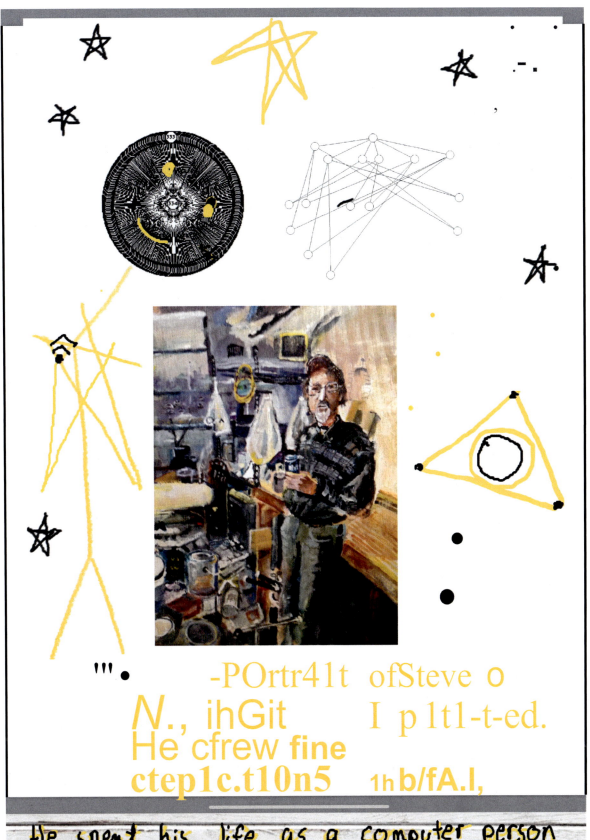

-POrtr41t ofSteve o N., ihGit I p1t1-t-ed. He cfrew fine ctep1c.t10n5 1h b/f A.I,

He spent his life as a computer person to become an artist late in life.

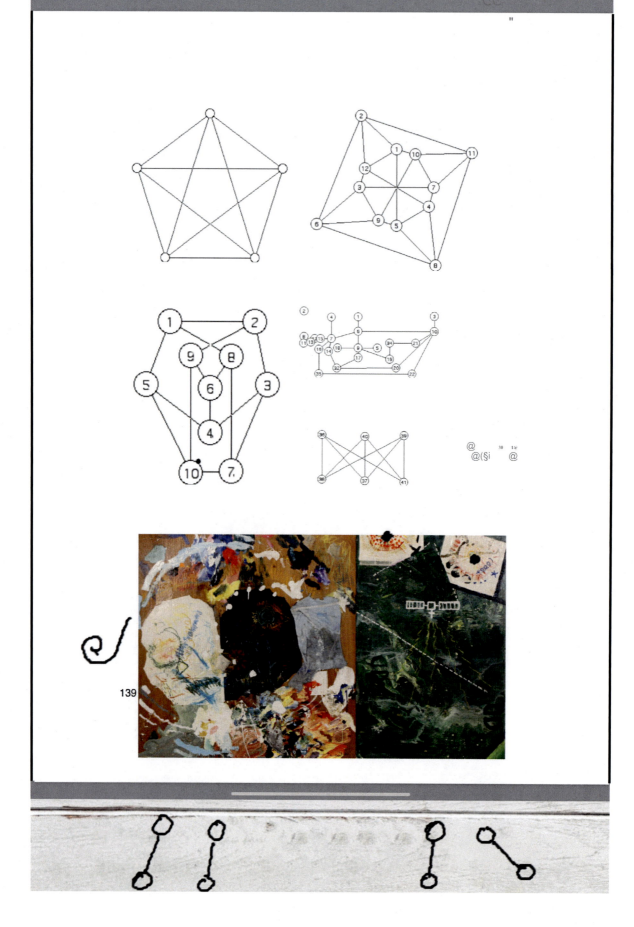

X

He can hardly get any air inside his lungs. His eyelids are blinking irregu larly. He plugs his ears while they pop as they wo uld at high altitudes. The pressures and tones lessen a little. The invisible weight lightens a littl e, and he can breath. A lunch bag is dropp ed inside the door. The symbols continue to flash. He stretches out his arm and can ju s t
bar e l y reach an orange in the brown bag. He rolls the orange on the floor and sm iles at its freedom .

> BRENT (VO.)
> The orange is free from pressure and can move?

SILENCE

Brent **Jlts** up and breathes deeply into the sile nce. He rubs his s hou ld ers, s tretchin g his neck. His attention returns to the orange. He bounces it off the walls, floor, and ceiling, findin g solace in a new kind of geometric repetition. He gets up with a new symbol in his hea d. He dra ws with his hand, a circle, and punctuates it with a dot in the middl e.
As he dra ws and punctuates the dot , he hears something in th e w all. The tones of periph ery sound soon return, followed by hyper-silence and excru ciating pressure.

> BRENT
>
> No you don' t.

This time, Brent sees an imaginary target on the wall. He throws the orange at it as hard as he can, like a *baseball* pitcher. It hits directly in the center of the wall and splats.
Pieces of orange drip down the wall to the floor. He stares at the crush ed orange for a long time.
<u>Brent eats from the pieces on the floor. The noises subside.</u>

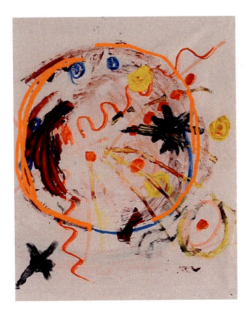

141

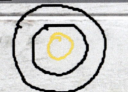

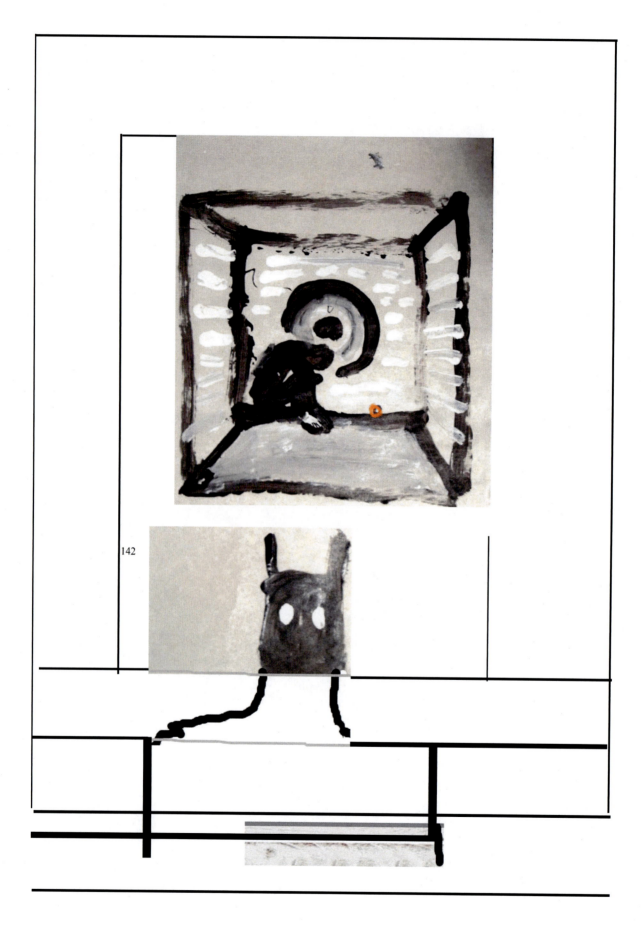

142

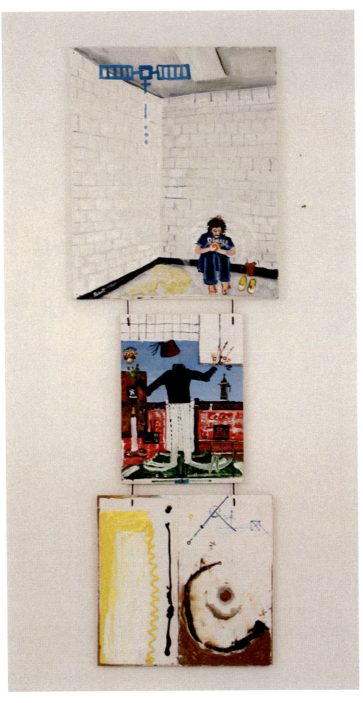

> BRE NT
> WHAT is the SOURCE?

> BRENT (VO.)
> The energy patterns? Why do I feel such sex ual energy and severe weight? This has got to stop.

> MALE VOICE (VO.)
> Brent?

Brent puts his ear to the wall, con fused from the defini te perso nal voice. He thinks he is hear in g throug h the wall. There is an undeniable and total silence.

> MALE VOICE (VO.) (voice is very faint)
> Brent .

> BRE NT (V.O .)
> I just h ea rd my name.

> BRE NT
> H ELLO!

> MALE VOICE (V O.)
> We think you can hear us?

Brent, a little spooked, looks around the room for a speaker; he even checks the vent. He puts his ear again, to the wall, thinking he was hearing soun d from the ad jo ining cell.

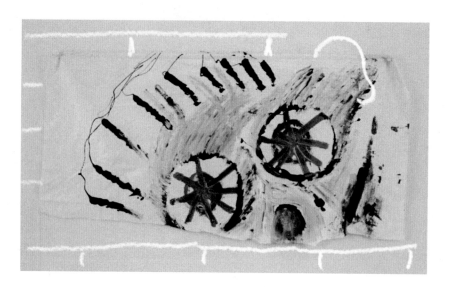

> BRENT *(yelling to the wall)*
> Anyone over there?! Can you hear me?

> MALE VOICE (V.O.)
> Brent, we are here. You can back away from the wall if you want. Focus in your mind.

Brent backs away from the wall.

> MALE VOICE (v.O.)
> Brent?

> BRENT (V.O.)
> There must be microphone s and speakers in the walls?

Brent checks the vents again.

> BRENT (V.O .)
> Brent? Who's "WE"?

> BRENT
> What? We? Who 's we? Who ARE you?

> BRENT (VO.)
> How I am I hearin g someone that I can't see, and ther e are no apparent speakers? It's NOT being projected from the wall. The relationship of distance from wall doesn' t matter; it's not any more loud, or any mor e quiet , based on distance. I am hearing in my mind more than with my ear.

> WISE WOMAN *(concerned voice)*
> Brent, we are here. We know you can't see us, but you have to trust us.

> BRENT
> Hold on, who is this? I just heard a voice in the wall?

> BRENT (V.O.)
> This jail is for men!?

WISE WOMAN (concerned voice)
Forget about the wall for now. We thought you'd never ask who we are!

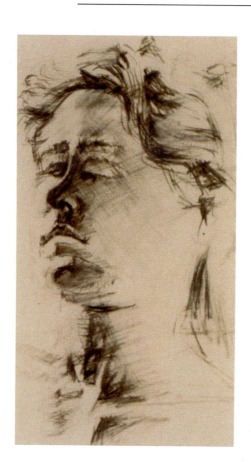

MALE VOTCE (V.O.)

Hey, Brent. This is incredible stuff. There are several of us monitoring you right now. My name is PETER. I am a man like you, just standing on the other side of a computer. It is good to finally meet you. I think our connection i wor king.

[APPLAUSE in the background.]

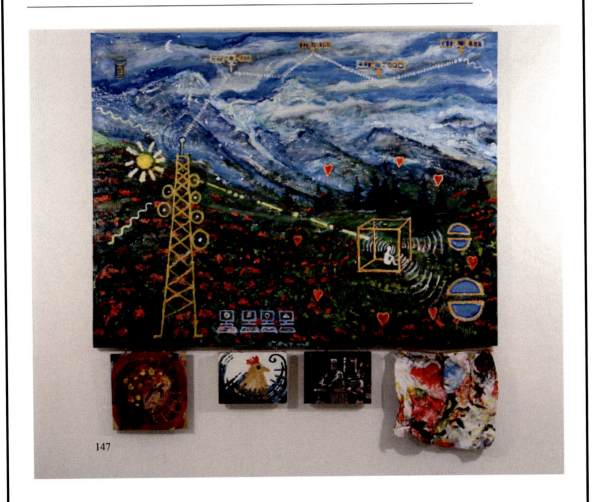

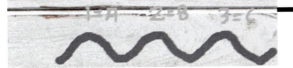

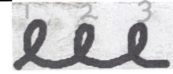

PETER (V.O.)
You have been through a hell of an experience.

BRENT
What the FUCK? Well, PETER *(sarcastically),* for "Pete's sake," what is going on?

BRENT (VO.) *(to himself)*
Nothing! My perception of REALITY is rapidly diminishing! My name is Brent Weston. Start there. I have some parents. My name is Brent. My name is Brent. My name is Brent.

PETER (V.O.)
BRENT TAPLIN WESTON, I'm going to overlook your first ques tion **, but just think** where you COULD be. **With that** aside, you may not think this possible, but you've been c01mected with us through a tower and satellites. Let's just say for now, you've entered a conversa tion wi th a pre tty high circle. If on ly you understood where you are standing, you would feel honored, humbled, and probably, scared. You really surprised us when your heartbeat counteracted the "red bird."

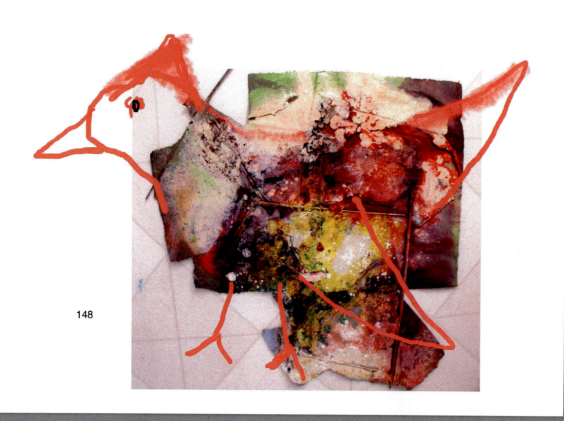

148

BRENT

Did I? Why? What tower? What birds are you talking about?

PETER (VO.)

What you thought sounded like a Cardinal. No one has ever so artfully... NOT succumbed to that sound.

BRENT (V O .) (to himself)

Brent! You remember the Cardinal. I thought the Cardinal sound was made by a man in a cell. He was trying to get my attention, and my gut said it was not a good situation. Blue bird= Okay.
Cardinal= Danger. Tower... There is one outside the jail. Is that it?

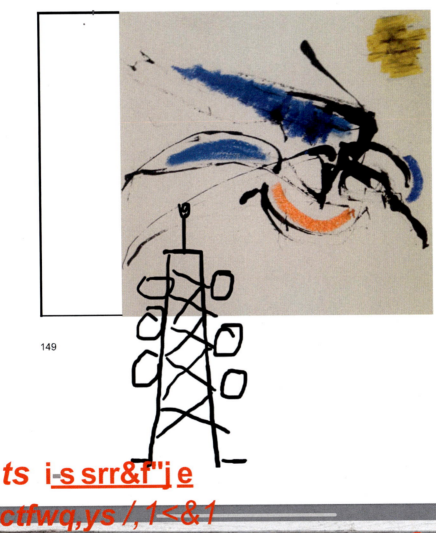

ts i-s srr&f"j e
ctfwq,ys /,1<&1
Th to cardinals.use I have

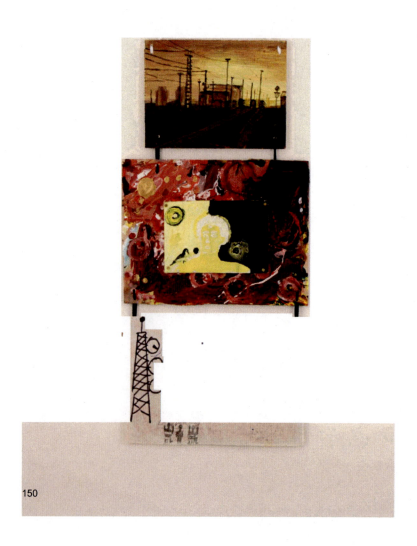

early conceptual drawing of what I thought was going on.

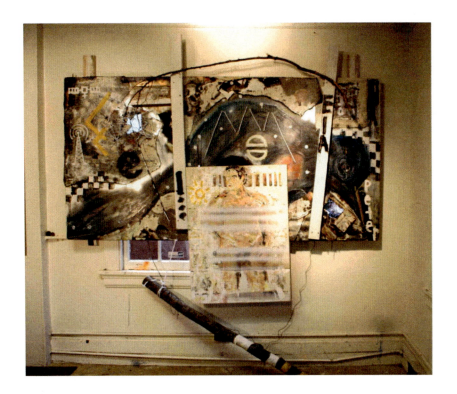

> PETER (VO.)
> We could tell you about the tower, but we won't, for now. Regarding your response to the red bird, it was pretty emotional for us as well!

Brent walks to the wall again and looks for speakers.

> PETER (V.O)
> Don't worry about any speakers, you won't be able to find them. However, the fact there are noises in the wall and floor is real.
>
> For now, concentrating on the wall actually takes attention away from how we commu nicate at thi s level. ln time, you will be able to decip her the di ffe rence be tter between modes of so und .

Tribute to the Bluebird

BRENT

IF I believe YOU, this will raise uncanny questions of reality. I'm already in a huge MESS! How would I know if it is you or God talking to me... my own self. And if its myself, what part? If there are parts?

PETER (VO.)
Always asking the tough questions first. Let's start with the practical.

WTSE WOMAN (VO.)
You have been up for days; you are wired and frazzled. You need to get some good rest.

PETER (VO.)
And Brent, we hate to be short, but getting some sound sleep is priority number one. There are also some initial protocols.

BRENT
Fuck protocol. I have questions. You owe me more knowledge than this.

[Long silence.]

BRENT
You there?

WTSE WOMAN (VO.)
Care to handle this one Pete?

PETER (V.O.)
Who me? *(laughs)* Not really, you go ahead.

WISE WOMAN
Maybe the best question right now Brent, is "Do you believe we **exist?**"

BRENT (VO.)
Shit! I don't know about y'all. BUT I EXIST! I am tired, extremely tired... that, I know. And I know my name *is* Brent! And my hand is bandaged... and bloody!

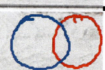

WTSE WOMAN (VO.)

Surprisingly, it is good for us to know with confidence, that you can recognize that. Why don't you try and get some sleep?

BRENT (VO.)

I would love to rest, okay? But every time I lie quietly, there are flashes of strange light and shapes, in my eyes. There are also strange tones and compressing pressures. And, what is going on with this hyper-sexual sensitivity I've got?

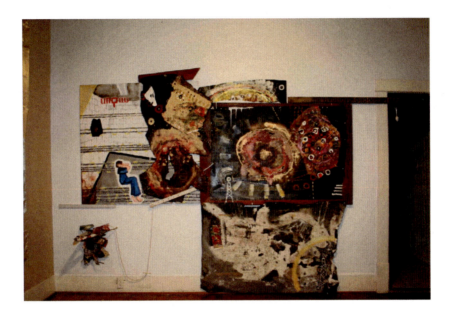

WISE WOMA N (V O.)
In time, Brent. We sympathize and have empathy for your right to be angry at this point, but NOW, you have to trust us. Try again, one more time, to get some sleep. We must run some tests, but
you should be able to get some sleep.

BRENT
Truth?

One piece of this painting escaped the fire.

> WTSE WOMAN (VO.)
> Yes.

> PETER (V O.)
> Have a little faith, son.

> BRENT
> Faith? My mind is shattered. I have a lot of questions, and I don't know how to even ask them anymore. And you ain't my dad!

> PETER (V O.)
> We will have plenty of time for this, BRENT.

Brent, almost in tears, curls up in the corner, tired beyond belief. He closes his eyes to merciful silence and gets some real sleep, possibly for the first time in days. It is the first time the whole jail building is at rest since he has been locked up. While asleep, Brent does not move in the slightest, and dreams that his brain is being mapped by a computer. His heartbeat seems influenced by the computer, and slows to a point that Brent thought dangerous even while sleeping. He awakens not knowing how long he

fl, Shade; of Oe'4th. (The Shadow of Death)
INT. WHITE CELL (SHADOW) ---------NIGHT

The air-conditioner jolts Brent awake, and he remembers the ensuing cold. He takes a moment to register his surroundings... a cell with windows to the lobby. He grins.

> BRENT
> At least they told the truth. I was able to get SOME sleep. The whole world seemed quiet.

He breathes in the silence.

Looking out the window, he sees a SHADOW move behind some blinds in an office at the back of the lobby. [A DOOR LOCKS, a GUN FIRES, a HAMMER POUNDS a nail.] Brent's body shakes violently with the sharp sounds. He now associates the hammer with Christ's crucifixion.

> BRENT (VO.)
> These sounds are evil. Not again. I just woke up.

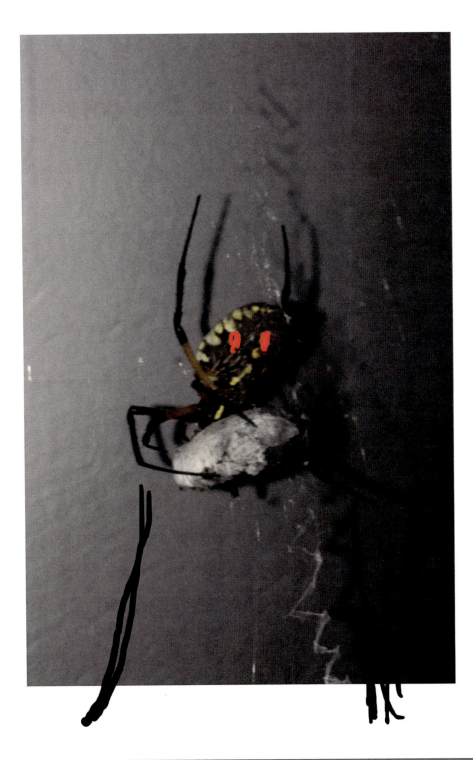

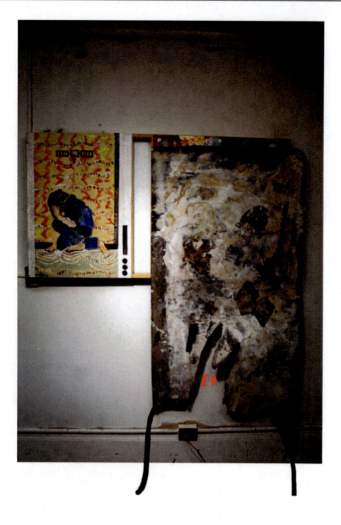

          BRE NT
        Peter. Are you there? Peter?

          BRE NT (v.0.)
        Peter? Oh my God, was that all a dream?

Brent hear s no signs of Peter, or anyone for that fact.

          BRENT
        Shit.

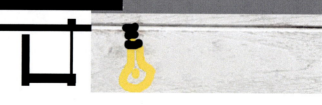

Brent is extremely cold. Brent looks back at the "Batman" shadow, and his face gets serious as he feels a kind of evil fall over the cell.

> BRENT
> PETER, where are you? I'M locked in a white cell, and its freezing cold.

Brent walks around the cell, then looks around at the shadow one more time. This time, the shadow appears to shift just a little, raising its right hand ever so slowly. Brent stares at the shadow. He hears Bach; Brent doesn't know much composition by Bach.

> BRENT (V.O.)
> This is spiritual, and there is evil coming from the room of that shadow. What are you? Why are your evil waves passing towards ME?

Brent hears the song *Shine*, by COLLECTIVE SOUL, playing very faintly in the background. It is louder than waking from deep slumber with a song stuck in mind. Brent goes down to the ground as a content deer, then gets up kneeling on one knee. Next, he stands up like a tree waving its "branches" dropping its fruit of oranges. Lastly, he stands in a position of the cross.

> BRENT (VO.)
> As the deer pants for the water brook, so my soul pants for Thee.

The shadow's hand continues to rise slowly, almost imperceptive.

> BRENT (V.O.)
> That's demonic. No joke. It could be some sort of alien, but the probability of an alien contact feeling that evil, is miniscule.

Brent continues to stare at the shadow through the windows as he starts to circle his cell.

> VOICE OF THE SHADOW (VO.) (in Brent's mind)
> Evil. You say I am evil? What about you? You fare no better. Hid from your mother. Lied to your sister. Cheated on your paper in college. Did not report all your income for your taxes.
> Irresponsible with your money... and do you really know how to love people?

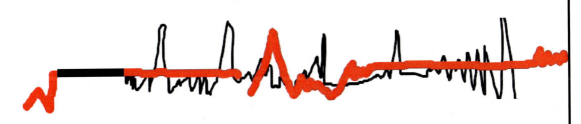

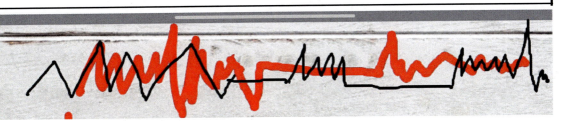

BRENT

That's almost **comical.** I was held accountable for the evil, but have you heard of redemption?

VOICE OF THE SHADOW (V.O.)
Bragged about your paintings. Cussed like a sailor. Jacked off for years. No faith in God. Life of doubt. You really don't know the goodness of God, do you!? TYU2360WOWYRosebowl-6-20-10

BRENT (V.O.)
PETER! Is this all tied into sound and the mind thing? Y'all will eventually use this worldwide? Ahh, shit.

BRENT (V.O.)
If it exists, it would first be used in privy circles and places of power. Can't go there!

VOICE OF THE SHADOW (V.O.)
And why NOT?

BRENT (V.O.)
There is someone much more powerful than privileged circles, YOU, and me. He suffered the consequences of my evil. Thanks to Him, I dance the dance of life.

VOICE OF THE SHADOW (VO.)
Shame. How you have been tricked!

Brent continues to feel evil pulsating in rings away from the shadow, attacking him. It is the scariest feeling Brent has ever felt. He begins to dance, repeating the formations of going to the ground like a deer, rising to one knee, standing as a tree dropping oranges, making a cross, and falling to the ground again. It is not the darks of shadow imagery that bothers Brent, but evil personified.

BRENT
You are wasting your time. In my entire, confusing life, this is the only thing I am absolutely sure of...

VOICE OF THE SHADOW (V.O.) (interrupting)
... Evil.

Brent feels mentally defeated for a brief moment. The *waves* of energy feel like total death. He rises and repeats his dance, over and over.

> BRENT (VO.)
> On rare occasions, the must intense feelings *have* been when I thought Evil was present, and common, everyday grace and goodness, gets lust. Dues evil actually exist at all, in any ultimate way?

Brent gives up and recoils on the ground in a fetal position. He feels as if he was in the womb of God, cocooned in a force field of grace emanating from each bodily lim b.
Something dramatic is happening all around him. It is a batt le of the cosmos. He is able to rest quietly, but this is only temporary.

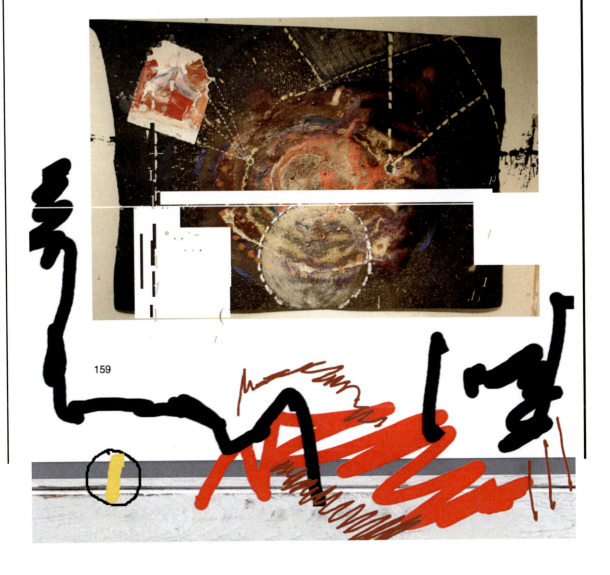

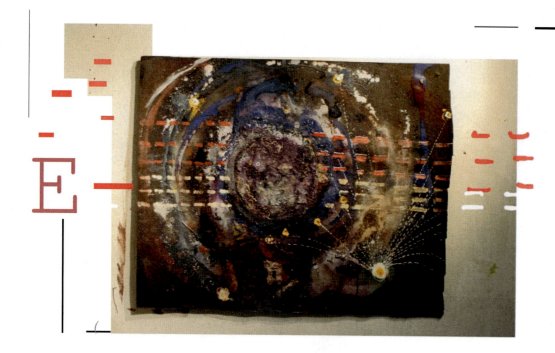
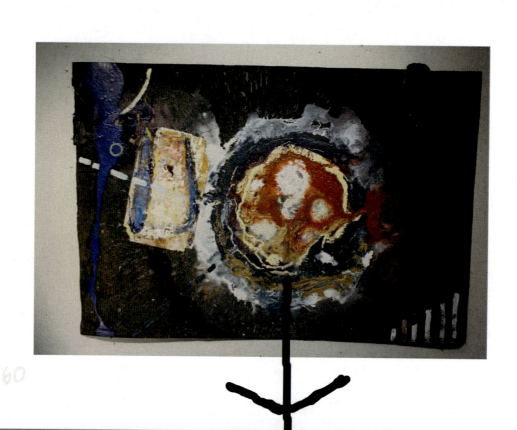

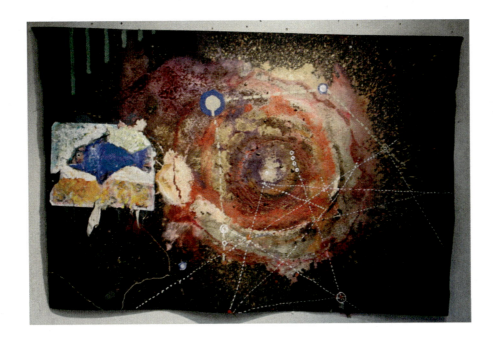
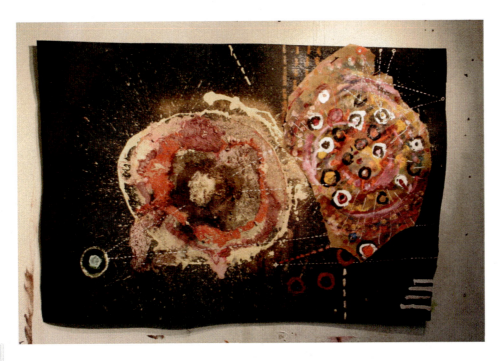

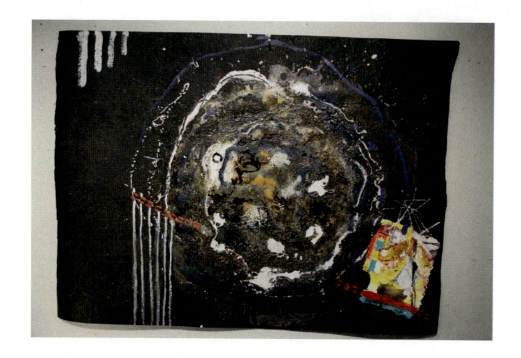

BRE NT (V O)
Something very wrong is passing over me . T KNOW real evil exists. Its waves are coming directly towards me. It is too strong to deny.

BRENT
Good MUST, and DOES exist as well! I'm DEAD without it.

Brent rises to one knee bowing his head.

BRENT (VO.)
The God T choose to serve is GOOD and forgiving. Evil will lose this battle for my soul. Even if you are the spirit of the Antichrist, you can't face the God of TRUTH who protects. You may take my life, but you won 't have my soul. The created is not stronger than the CREATOR of the w1iverse. It is to the Creator, I bow and trust.

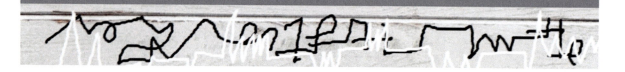

> BRENT
> What are you? You are but me rely a created being.

> VOICE OF THE SHADOW (V.O.)
> You don't even know if I'm a god or godde88.

> BRENT
> You are just a created being.

> BRENT (v. O.)
> T need to talk to E about this.

> UNKNOWN VOICE (from the deep)
> Her doubts are not yours.

> VOICE OF THE SHADOW (VO.)
> You don't know if I'm real, or an illusion.

> BRE NT
> Screw you! You are talking to me. YOU are aliv e, and I'M alive. lam ...
> REAL!

The shadow remains, but the presence of evil is diminishing.

> BRENT
> The God of Truth protects me. You had your choice, just like the rest of us. And what did you choose?

The shadow's hand slowly stops moving.

> BRENT (w ith tears and au thori ty)
> You turned your back on the love, grace, and goodness of your Creator. *(sincere and compassionate)* I am sorry.

> VOICE OF THE SHADOW (VO.)
> There i8 a new battle that ha8 ju8t begun in thi8 world. If you uniy understood. You already have the mark.

Brent looks at the top of his right hand, bandaged and bloody.

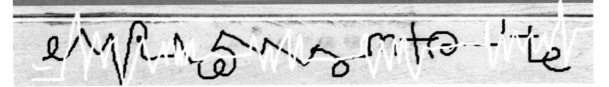

BRENT (V.O.)

That's a wound. It will heal and leave a scar. Maybe a reminder of what is to come, and that I have a choice.

VOICE OF THE SHADOW (V.O.)

Choice, you think people have a choice. If the goodness of God is all that you know, where is any choice? And why does a GOOD God even allow for evil?

BRE N T

Rea l questions, they are, but not for a fini te mind. Take it up with your Crea tor, IF YOU CAN! You were once really beau tifu l, weren't you?

Brent spins around and around with his hands out like a cross. From above, it looks like a red circle has been drawn around him. The core middle is navy blue. The circle turns

It. The Ftya;1 e Z ,t WiQppir,+l\e 8'1QCl.....lc,'ltf.rfhiS

INT. WHITE CELL (FLY) ------------NIGHT

~~Brent sits down and immediately a FLY~~ enter s the room. Its organic buzzing lays a blanket of peace across Brent's shoulders. Relaxed, refreshed, quick as lightening, Brent catches the fly in his hand .

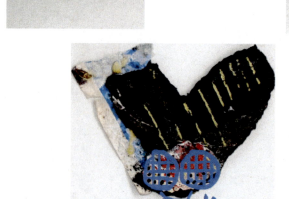

w s   Friend.

>   BRENT
>   Hello, my little friend! Up for a game of catch?

Brent opens his hand. The fly buzzes and zigzags in front of Brent's face. Brent catches him with his left hand.

>   BRENT
>   Left handed. I AM good.

Brent opens his hand, and the fly loops around Brent's head and pauses in front of Brent's forehead. Brent's hand whips up to his head. Fly drops to Brent's waist and then his knees. Brent's hand comes up empty.

>   BRENT (VO.)
>   Little friend, I feel like the Holy Spirit has been upon you. Thank you for somehow getting into this locked room inside the middle of the jail.

The fly heads under the door and leaves. Brent shivers with freezing cold. He lies on the mat that was thrown into his cell. He rests in peace for a few minutes. Brent has his eyes shut for a few moments.

INT. WHITECELL (MAT) --------NIGHT

>   PETER (VO.)
>   Brent, we think we've got back on line.
>
>   BRENT
>   Ahhh, NO!

Brent sits up.

>   BRENT
>   You missed out on the party! Where have YOU been?

There is no answer.

>   BRENT
>   Are you there?

Tmm edia tely.

> PETER (V.O .)
> Yes, Brent. Look inside the mat.

> BRE N T
> You have to be kidding me. What just happened? I just saw a demon, or the spirit of the Antichrist, with my eyes.

> PETER (VO.)
> Just look inside the mat.

Brent tears open a comer of the mat.

> PETER (VO.)
> Pull out the stuffing to the mat.

He pulls out all the stuffing. A "ZEST" soap wrappe r falls to the floor.

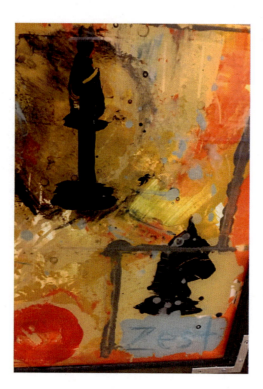

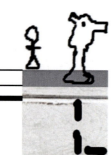
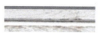
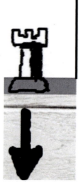

BRENT (V.O.)
Color! It's a kind of small painting, of sorts.

PETER (V.O.)
Do those letters mean anything to you?

BRENT (VO.)
Yes, "ZEST" = NEST. And the simple fact of colors in a white cube.
Thank you, Peter.

Tears flo w.

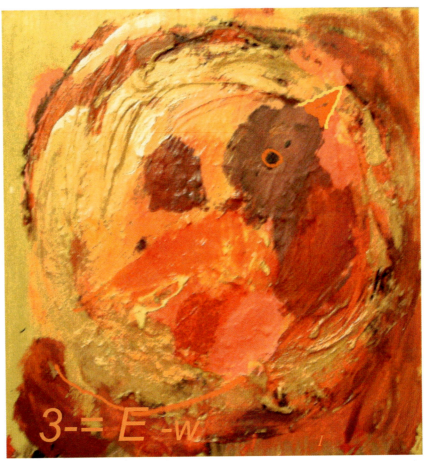

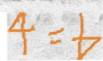

r_..

J,.

...

e a.

e1a

4

-

h 1. The word "Op," was totally added to the cover by OCR. Of all the words on the planet, it chose that one. P is also the 16th letter of the alphabet. The number 6, I have always associated with the letter b. The letter "b" is the lower case of my first initial. Substitute the "16" with "1b" for the "p" and you get "O1b" or "O1B" for the word "Op." Rearrange the letters and you get OB1. If you this think this is strange, it is the way I interpret. It is weird. There is another correction on the cover, that is more immediately specific, and has a "back channel" to the story. It's a game changer. I chose to leave it a mystery.

Pd
i!   O m
E - 3 -w
     O
Un

        PETER (V.O .)
        You are welcome, Brent.

        BRENT (VO.)
        But I want to know what happened back there with the shadow.

INT. WHITE CELL (BEACH CONVERSATION) -------------NIGHT

        PETER (V O .)
        Sit down amongst the stuffing. Just pretend you are on the beach for the fun of it. Get your mind out of the cell for a minute.

Brent builds himself a little nest of stuffing on his pretend beach, and leans up against the wall.

        BRENT
        This ain't no beach.

        PETER (V.O.)
        No, it's not. But just relax. There are a few things I want to share with you, so RELAX.

        BRENT
        I'm all ears, what's left of them.

        PETER (VO.)
        With the shadow, in simple language, you blew the circuit and "beat" the computer. To boot, you MAY have seen some sort of vision. You were experiencing the possible evil of new, sound and mind, technology. You saw firsthand how it can affect the world. In fact, you really scared some people. The intensity of your experience convinced some of us that you were dealing with more than just a big computer program. Some of us thought you were dealing with the spirit behind the programs. Those on our end who are Christians, have a different take on what happened than those of our closest friends and colleagues . It's worldview versus worldview, and you maintained, at some level, that the Personal and Spiritual was created in this universe by a Good God .
        Brent, it is important for you to know that people have given their lives for the technologies you now know of, spirit or no spirit! I

say this not to frighten you. In time, you will learn how to wisely deal with what you have been given, and what will be thrown your way. Do you understand? And by the way, the epistemology you learned at L'Abri... you may, or may not, remember drawing on the wall... good stuff.

[Long pause]

BRENT (VO.)
Why was I drawing epistemological substratum on the wall? don't really remember much of that from L'Abri. Are you referring to *f's* subject-object-criteria triangle . Wasn't God in the middle, giving meaning to the broken, three focal points?

PETER (VO.)
You spun the triangle and formed a dynamic circle and sphere. Apparently, God's Spirit spoke to you even through an imperfect epistemology. The epistemological tool reminded you of your presence in this world.

BRENT (VO.)
I never really understood J's epistemology, though I felt like God was with me. Look Peter, I am scared I'm a prophet in the end time scenario. I don't think I could ever go to Israel.

PETER (V O.)
Why?

BRENT (V.O .)
This all could go to my head as a Messiah complex . I'm already struggling with that. The way the religious right uses *Revelation* to scare people into "salvation," **REALLY** bothers me! Some people are more worried about the "Second Coming" than the living Christ in the rest of Scripture.

Peter is quiet. Brent feels like a child and creates a flat dove from the mat's shtffing. He slides it into the middle of the room. The dove is about a foot in circumference.

INT. WHITE CELLCONVERSATION (BUTTERFLIES)--------------NIGHT

Brent notices a pamphlet pushed under the door. It is the rules of the jail, and the rights

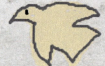

of inmate s. Brent is completel y unable to focus and read them, as his eyes seem scrambled too much for the small writing. He tears the pamphlet into three pieces. He fidgets with them during conversation.

> PETER (V O.)
> Brent, we would like your advice for the future of our satellites. How many do you want? Also, if you had to assemble a team of advisors, who would they be?
>
> BRE N T (VO.)
> How many satell ites do **T** want? What? What a weird and strange question. *(pause, Brent laughs)* You are losing my confidence that you exist.
>
> PETER (VO.)
> This is no jok e.
>
> BRENT
> Okay, I will take three. What are they used for? Concerning the team, that would not be difficult.
>
> PETER (VO.)
> Before I answer YOUR question , let's try something. We want you to stop talking out loud. You have been on our radar for awhile. Imperfect as it is, we have an idea to your thoughts, a link of sorts.
>
> BRENT (VO.)
> How deep into my consciousness... subcon sciousness?
>
> PETER (V.O .)
> It gets tricky, fast, especially the deeper we go.
>
> BRE N T (V O .)
> I can understand how I may be able to hear you, a super high or low frequency, but how do you read my thoughts?
>
> PETER (VO.)
> Brent, unfortunately I am not allowed to talk much about this with you. You can call it protocol.

let me take some of the punches

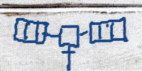 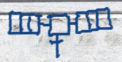 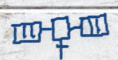

BRENT
Handy for you, ain't it.

PETER (V.O.)
I suppose, but believe me, I don't know about all the science, either. I can tell you that some things can be inversely read.

BRENT
What the hell does that mean?

PETER (VO.)
Strike two; try THINKING the thought.

BRENT (VO.)
This ain't baseball.

PETER (VO.)
You sure?

BRENT (raises his voice and smiles)
Non capisco! And you know I'm going to strike out. I stunk at baseball in high-school.

PETER (V.O)
Funny.

BRENT (V.O.)
I thought so.

PETER (VO.)
You are catching on.

BRENT (VO)
To change subjects, are you a Christian? You said, "Those of us," earlier. I only ask because I need to be able to trust anyone that has access to my mind.

PETER (VO.)
Interesting you asked. Yes, I am. Maybe a different flavor, but yes. However, for the rest of your life, you will be dealing with people that are, and more often, are not. I was chosen to
speak with you first because of my understanding of your past.

BRENT (VO)
Why do I get the impression you are African American?

PETER (VO.)
Because I AM black.

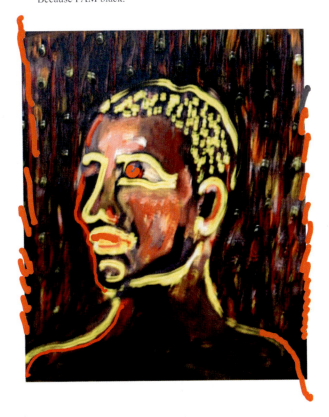

BRENT (V.O.)
How did I know that?

PETER (V.O.)
Top secret.

BRENT (VO.)
Howdidl endupinhere?

PETER (VO)
Like your physics classes, you may never understand it.

BRENT (VO.)
Low blow!

PETER (VO)
What happened to you in the GA TECH physics classes?

BRENT (loudly)
T FATLED. Several times!

PETER (VO)
Stepping out to "bat" again.

BRENT(VO.)
"Hit batsman ."

PETER (V.O.)
Believe me, we already know you failed physics.

[Pause]

BRENT (VO.)
I liked studying the physics of PING PONG, more than learning formulas. Then after my travels, I really was an ARTIST.

[Pause]

PETER (VO.)
Physics is an art too, Brent.

BRENT (smiling)
MAYBE?

PETER (VO.) (laughing)
Anyway, Europe was good to you! Milking cows on the tops of the Swiss Alps... painting on the streets of Europe... L'Abri...

Rand J... Monzambano, Morocco, Ronchamp... the Hagia Sophia.

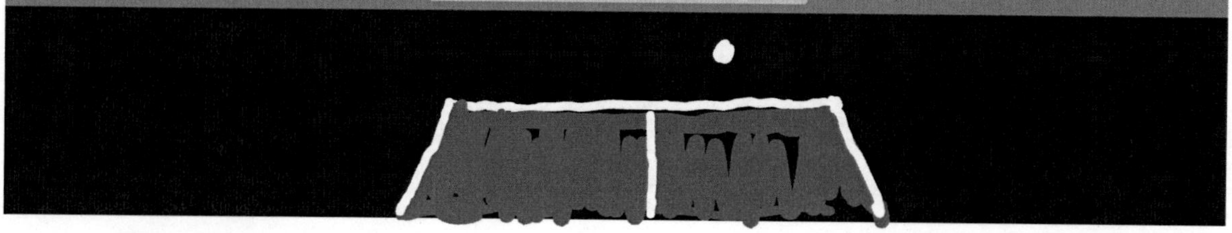

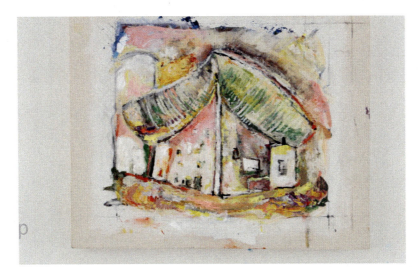

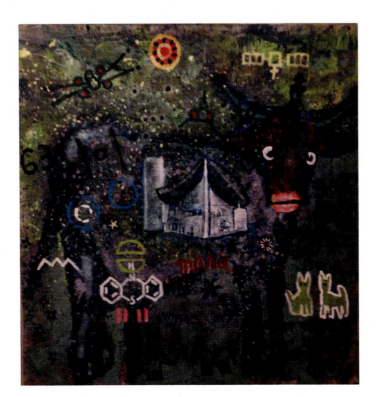

One of my FAVORITE Pieces of Architecture

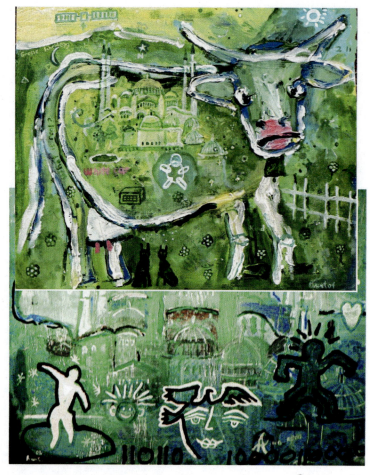

(Y\qd,e *0-..* pil8rirr. it. to+ha. Soir. So phi   t',
IsfQI'\'o-,l. Pl°""e. hciJ *4c* ""C{lle *eme'{*

Thank you Prof Jones for encouraging me to GO

BRENT (VO.)
Not much you don't already know about me.

PETER (VO.)
I particularly like the light at Corfu.

BRENT (VO)
That was one of the simplest drawings in my journal.

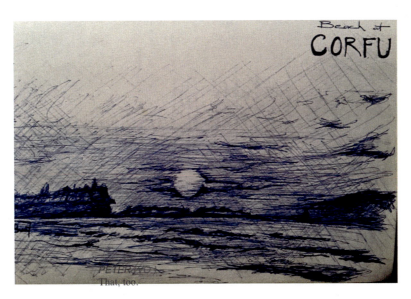

PETER (VO.)
That, too.

Brent starts folding the pieces of the pamphlet into three origami butterflies.

PETER (V O.)
Where would you like those satellites?

BRENT (VO.)
What did you say they would be used for?

PETER (V.O.)
The word "satellite" will mean more to you as time passes. know you need to relieve yourself, and the guards have not opened the door when you knocked. They are coming for you in a little while, but if you can't wait that long, feel free to use the floor.

BRENT (VO)
I'll definitel y have me a beach, then.

[Pause]

BRENT (VO)
It just won't be at Corfu.

BRENT (VO.)
Okay, besides satellites in the U.S. of A.?

PETER (V.O.)
Yes.

BRENT (VO.)
Australia, the Middle East, and Switzerland.

PETER (V O)
Thank s, I'll pass this on.

BRENT (VO)
Peter, you know that stuff doesn't intere st me right now. Am l going to see *E* again?

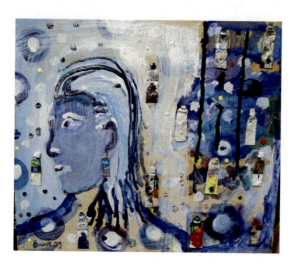

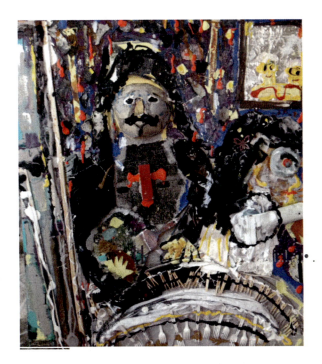

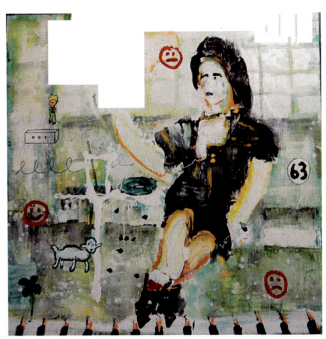

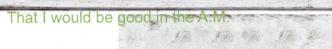

That I would be good in the A.M.

PETER (V O.)
I can't answer that, but I will tell you she's moving to California like she said she might. We know you would have died for her. Be prepared to let the thought of being with her die as well. You must face the fact that she will probably never marry you.

BRENT (VO)
Great. I wonder if there may be a huge earthquake in Californi a.

PETER (VO.)
Why do you thi nk that?

BRENT (VO)
It's a long story, and that journal is now gone.

PETER (V O.)
We can discuss the diary poem of the rams and earthquake, later. Hopefully, we will have a lot of time.

BRE N T
You couldn't possibly read my mind back then! Brent

has finished making his butterflies. He sits back against the wall.

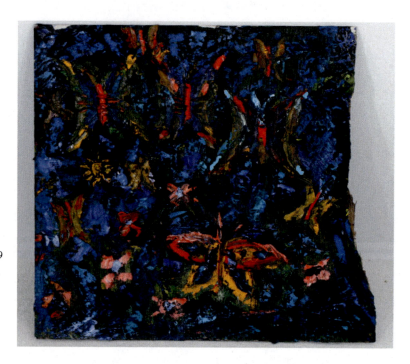

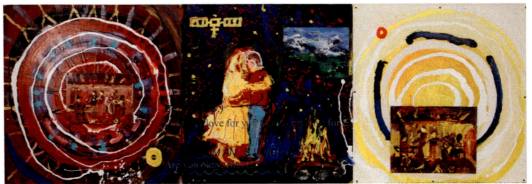

                    BRENT
                    Who are you?

                    PETER (V.O.)
                    She is a good friend. And remember, you do not need to respond out
                    loud... baseball.

                    WISE WOMAN'S VOICE (V O.)
                    Thank you, Peter.

Brent smiles.

                    WISE WOMAN'S VOICE (VO.)
                    I am a Christian psychologist that has been studying your case. This
                    is a pretty awesome event. You have quite a history .

                    BRENT (V O.)
                    If you only knew.

                    WISE WOMAN'S VOICE (VO.)
                    I know more, and less, than you think I know, but I certainly
                    know details about your past, and a little about HOW you think.
                    You have recently been through some tough times. Are

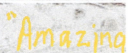 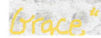

you relatively okay, now? It seems to us you have reached a lucid pocket after a "re-birthing."

BRENT (VO.)
Are you here to counsel me on E?

WISE WOMAN'S VOICE (VO.)
If that is what you want.

BRENT (VO)
I love her!

WISE WOMAN'S VOICE (VO.)
That has been established. You think you can live without her?

BRENT (VO.)
Hell, I don't know.

WISE WOMAN'S VOICE (V.O.)
Honestly, it's going to be tough!

BRENT (VO) *(sarcastically)*
Only thought the wedding held nationwide interest.

WISE WOMAN'S VOICE (VO.)
It's not ALL been your doing. Don't be too hard on yourself.

BRENT (VO.)
I'll always have a special place for her down deep.

WISE WOMAN'S VOICE (V.O.)
Yes.

Brent slides one of the butterflies under the door.

BRENT
I -

Brent slides another under.

>   *BRENT*
>   Am -

And another.

>   *BRENT*
>   Fine.

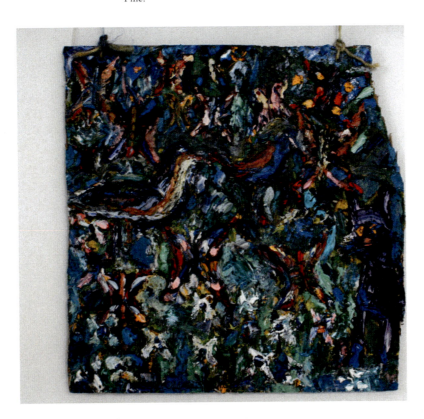

>   Brent, there are some things we need to briefly talk about.
>
>   *BRENT (VO.)*
>   I rememb er, baseball!

WISE WOMAN'S VOICE (VO.)
No, but glad you remember. Your status is that you are still in jail. There is no "Get out of jail free" card. This is no picnic. Your parents cannot currently pay bond, and you are currently on record for a felony.

BRENT (VO.)
Well, I've got you and Peter, and whomever else is behind the curtain. I think I need TOTO.

WISE WOMAN'S VOICE (VO.)
Dogs are good, but like J said, you are still in jail, and the time may come when you will forget and doubt us.

BRENT (VO.)
You must be joking.

WISE WOMAN'S VOICE (V.O.)
No. Just be you, and you will make it.

Through the window in his cell, Brent sees a group of men and women staring in at him. He hears them talking.

MAN #1
So, the film's climax is his dance and fight with the evil shadow.

MAN #2
We should be completely free with it, no inhibitions. Let that scene take us wherever it will.

MAN #1
And if it's long, we let it run long.

BRENT (VO.)
Movie? You must be shitting me. Are y'all hearing this, too? Come on computer people, talk to me!

Some people on the other side of the window are crying, looking into his cell.

BRENT (VO.)
There's no way to capture on film the evil intensity. It was not the shadow as much as the SPIRIT. It would come across as a joke.

> MAN #1
> We will need to use all the tricks, the right music...

Brent has heard all he needs to hear, then pees and craps on the floor near the stuffing.

> BRENT
> I now have a BEACH, you pricks.

INT. WHITE CELL ---------MORNING?

Guards A and B open Brent's door and step inside.

> GUARD A *(African American)*
> Let's go!

Brent doesn't move.

> GUARD B *(White)*
> You are switching rooms, kid. Get up.

Brent doesn't move.

> BRENT (V.O.) *(looking at GUARD A)*
> One good guard, *(looking at GUARD B)* and one bad guard.

Guard A takes his hands. Guard B takes his feet, and they haul him into another cell.

13. The -1 oAf He

1!

lEc

They dump Brent into a small room with gray walls and Plexi-glass windows. Brent feels a different, overwhelming evil return. He shivers uncontrollably and violently in the freezing room. His body temperature is all messed up. Brent's mind now feels totally scrambled, and his body jerks with each sharp sound. Thoughts, even to Brent, don't seem coherent.

> BRENT (V.O.)
> As Christians, we are to be like the lion, Asian, in *The Lion, the Witch, and the Wardrobe,* though my death will atone for no one. This is where I am going to die, in the service of Christ. My body and mind can take no more. I don't get a stone table, just the

concrete floor. I'm not too thrilled to have Dan Rather, the US military, and the whole world watching me die.

        BRENT
        Peter!

[Silence except for loud, sharp, clap noises.] Brent lies down; the pressures have returned. He is spread eagle on the floor. [HEART BEATING irregularly] He grins at what he sees - A CORDED STRING. It is the only loose thing in the cell. He is barely able to tie it around his left ring finger. Brent does this in memory of *E,* and is happy. Then he notices constellation maps in the spots on the floor.

        BRENT
        I'll draw Orion and the Big Dipper. Yes, yes... wait................*move* the North Star a little to the left.......perfect.

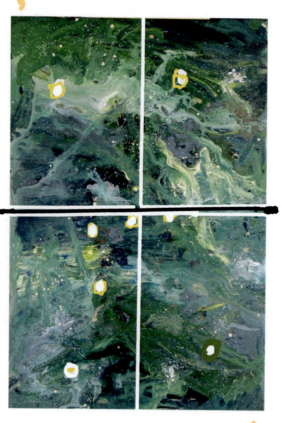

185

LJkere.

the streets have no name

[The constellation maps dissolve, and a star-filled, night sky evolves on the floor. The sky dissolves into the cell's original floor.]

INT. GRAY CELL----------NIGHT

Guard A enters the cell carrying a tray with a carton of milk, a cup of something, some grits, toast, a napkin, and a spoon. He places the tray on the ground and then exits.
Brent arranges his milk carton, cup and spoon, and napkins, in a circle. Guard A re enters and looks at Brent's arrangement.

> GUARD A
> You don't have it right.

The guard exits. Brent rearranges the configuration. The guard re-enters.

> GUARD A
> You still don't have it correct.

Brent rearranges the configuration in a square-like grid. Guards re-enter.

> GUARD A
> You haven't figured it out, have you?

Brent rearranges the configuration, trying, like it is the key to his survival. Guards re enter again.

> GUARD A to GUARD B
> He's not eating.

> BRENT
> Would you eat this stuff? I am not sure what arrangement code will get me out of this cell.

The guards are surprised by the question.

> GUARD B to GUARD A
> This boy's gonna make president.

They exit. Now, Brent is even more confused. Locked in his own mind, he recalls a conversation from the guards about medication and food.

in all four corners.

BRENT (V.O.)

Medication, that's the first time I've heard anything about that word.

Brent drinks from the carton and continues to move the tray items around and around.

BRENT (yelling)
I need to go to the restroom!

BRENT
PETER?! I need ya now, like "PRONTO!"

There is silence. He briefly pulls down his pants half way. Later, Brent is curled up in the center of the floor, shivering. Each little noise makes him jump almost in physical pain. Guard A opens Brent's door, retrieves the tray, and eyes Brent's refuse on the floor

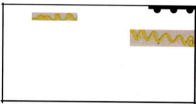

GUARD A
Clean that up, now.

BRENT (sarcastically)
Yes sir! How?!

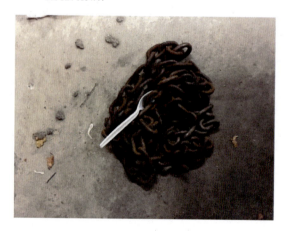

> GUARD A
> Fig ure it out!

The guard watches as Brent scoops his feces into the milk carton with a plastic spoon . Brent checks his pocket and wonders where his old spoon has gone.

> BRENT
> Ahh. Where 's MY spoon???

> BRENT (VO.)
> Must have had to turn it in when they ban dag ed my hand . Oh yeah, the security guard smiled when I gave it to him.

A new association with a white plastic spoon contradicts the jo yful memories. Brent places the carton on the tray. The guard carries it away. Through a window, he sees an inmat e in the adjoining cell stick a sin gle match into the key hole between cells.

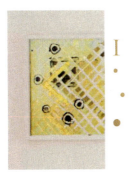
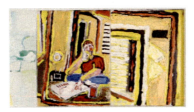

On the other side of th e cell is a steel, mesh door. On the door, is painted two pyra mids that connect and are sideways. They are yellow. Brent ha s never seen such a symbol. He looks through the mesh. In the door across the hall, is a window. Brent sees the backs of white-hooded people. They are facing a stage and are watching a woman in a flesh colored leotard sitting Indian style, doing yoga.

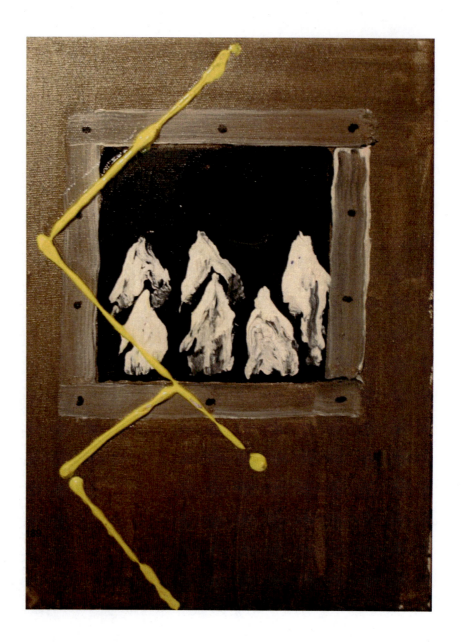

literally   'r\   t\e.((

 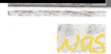

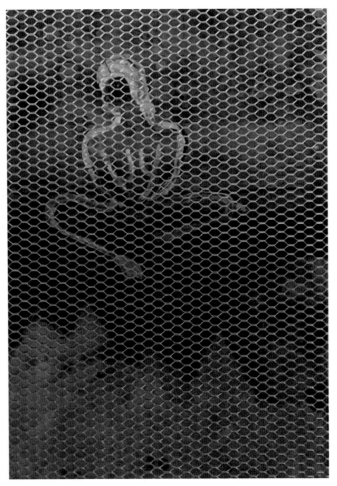

BRENT (V.O.)
What the hell? Are the old rumors of this jail being run by a KKK family, true? Is that lady real, or is she a projection on a screen?

Brent smashes his body up against the cell door, shaking.

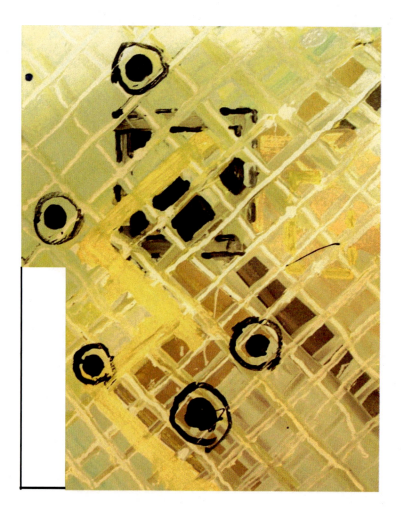

He starts to pull down his pants, but thinks better of it. He realizes that through all the sexual energy during the week, he has not masturbated and is content to wait. He looks at the string, turns away from the door, shuts his eyes, and makes hand signals in front of his face.

With or without you.

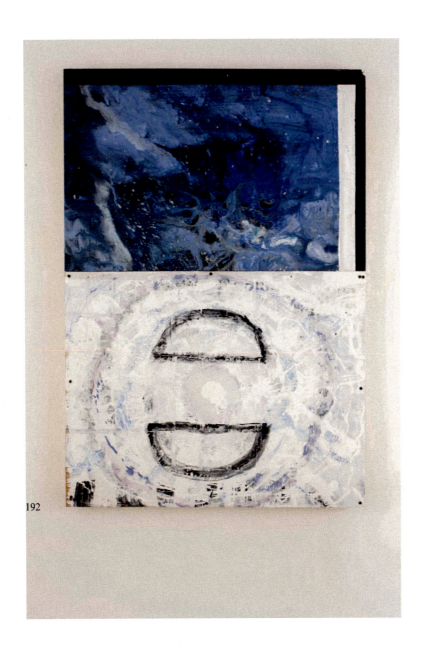

Pictures of You

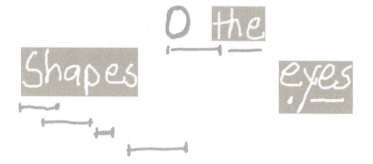

Ar.the Cure

The geome tric pa ttern s in his mjnd have returned.

ρ.. e 5

1

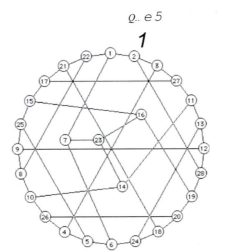

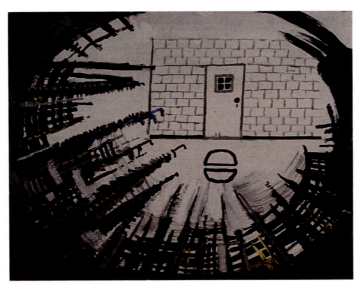

''
•

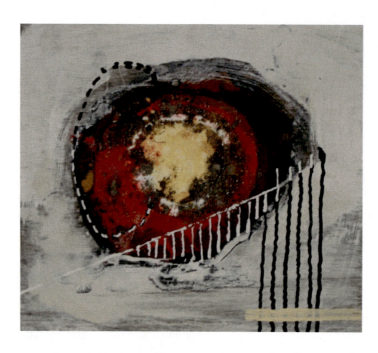

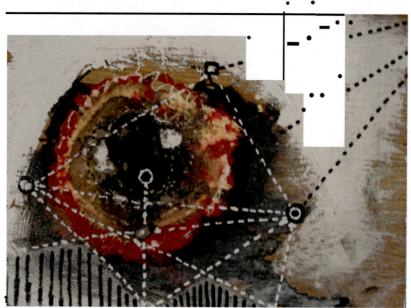

Intensity   the

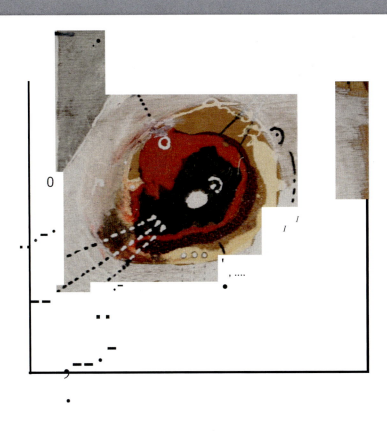

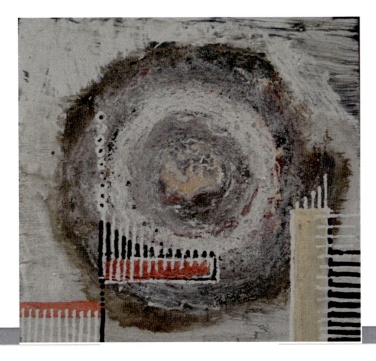

195

WT SE U NKNOWN VOTCE (V O .)
 Brent, we have to test these images in your current mental state, and we need to know if you would physically fight for a just and righteous cause?

BRENT (V O.)
Fuck you. I'll practice to disarm someone, but not take a life.

Brent touches his ear and continues making hand signals, which turn into a poor displ ay of martial arts. He does not know if the voices are real, anymor e. Tones and pressure nois es re tu rn, crushing him to the floor.

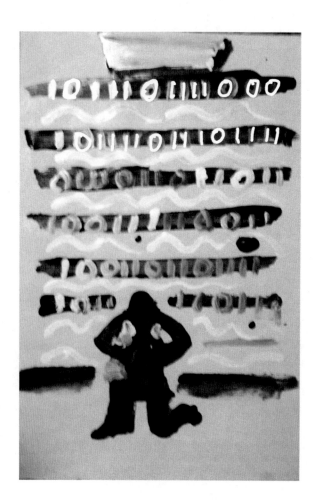

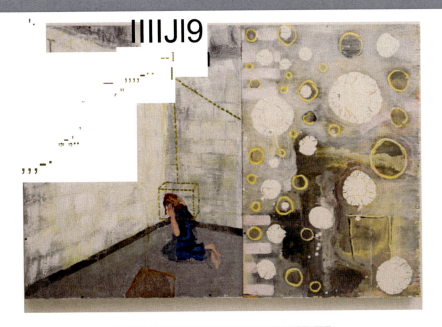

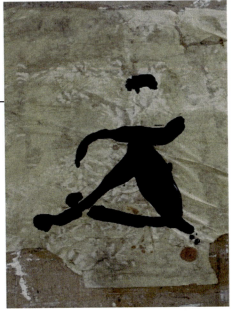

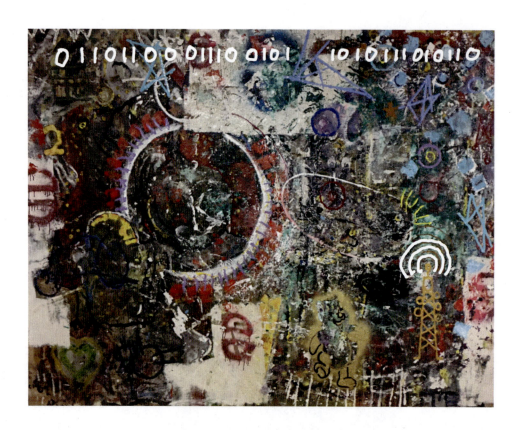
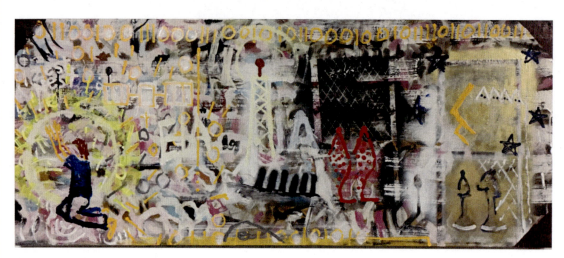

I noze

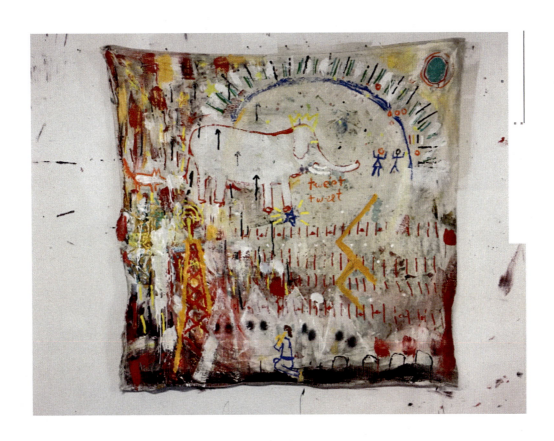
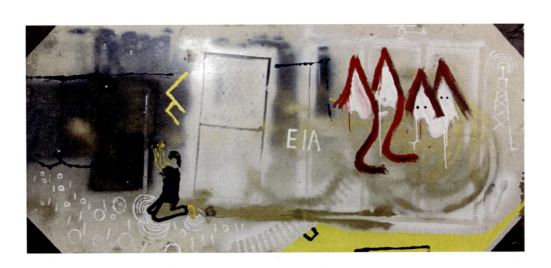

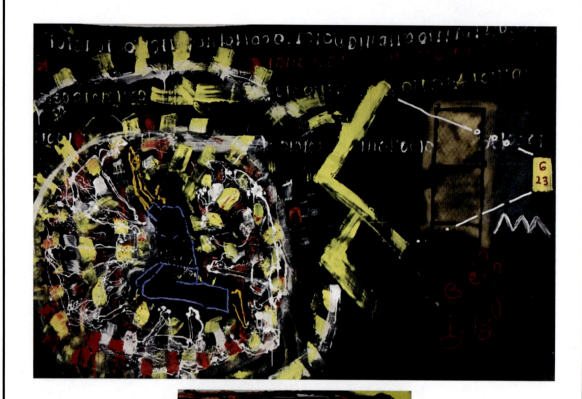

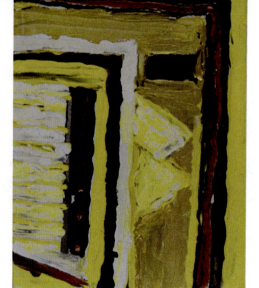

200

momant of surrender

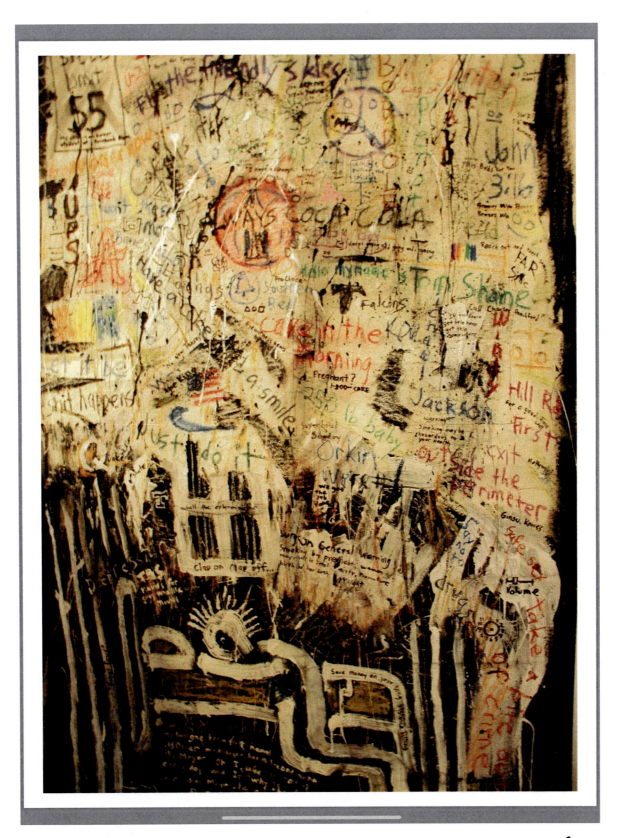

Manically painted from memory of commercials

Someone covers the window on the door across the hall, like a window on a ship. He feels cold enough that he could die. Any noise makes him jerk. Brent believes he will have to fight from cell to cell to stay alive, like in an underground Dungeon and Dragon's game; this becomes the breaking point.

     BRENT (V.O.)
    I can't fight anymore.

Rolling on the ground.

     BRENT (screaming in anguish)
    Jesssus! Help me!

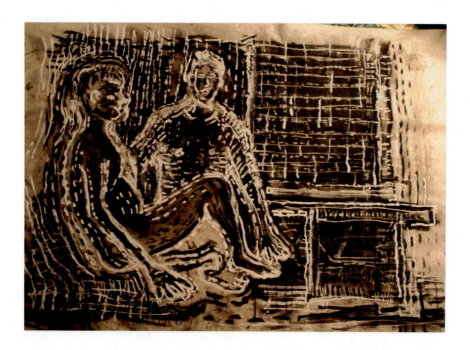

    Where am I? Am I literally, in hell? I have been totally forsaken.
    Where is the God from my childhood? I'm alone in

death, and none of my friends even know where I am. Each person that goes by is an intense, spiritual being.

Emotions are out of control, and then a return to a brief, stubborn lucidity. Praying...

> BRENT (V.O.)
> I still believe in Your mercy and that You created me with purpose.
> If I am left here for eternity, You are STILL my God.

An African American SHERIFF marches by the steel, mesh door.

> SHERIFF (ven; authoritatively, almost militaristic)
> MY NAME IS JESUS!

> BRENT (VO.)
> Why would a sheriff say that?

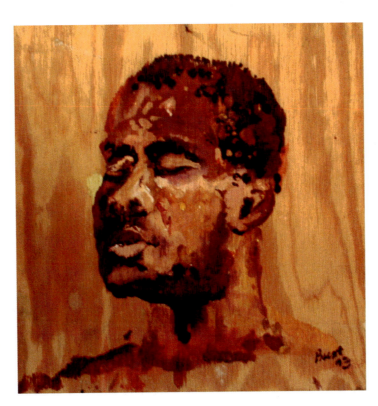

Brent closes his eyes and covers his ears.
[Brent becomes a Bishop, combined with a Knight, on a marble chess board.] [A hand moves the Bishop / Knight across the board.]
Later, a hand opens the door to Brent's cell. A hand opens the door to a police car. Brent sees sunlight for the first time in days.

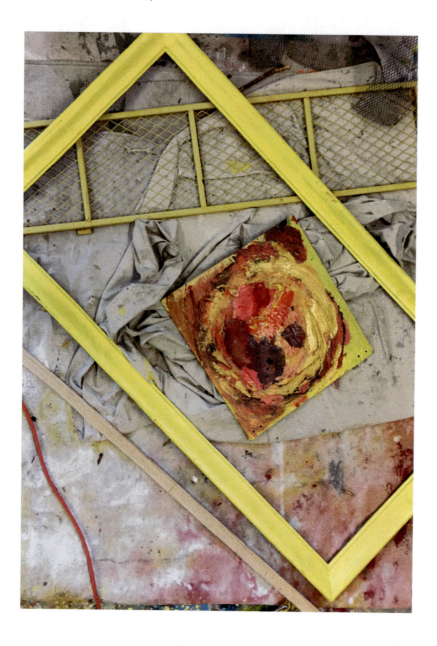

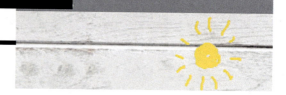

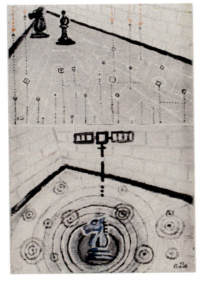
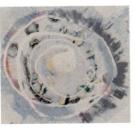
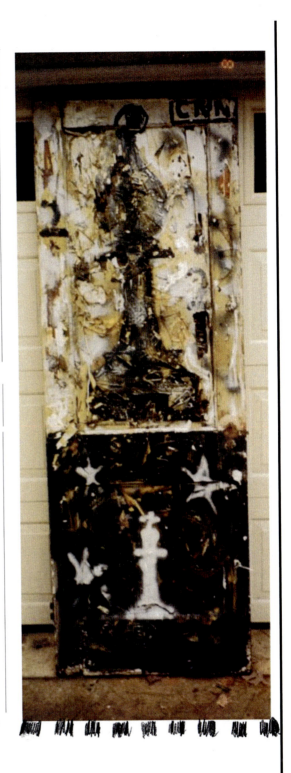

we

Is my story fake too?

INT. POLICE CAR ----------DAY

Brent opens his eyes and finds himself inside a police car. The policeman's radio crackles with chatter. Brent presses his nose slightly against the window. The sheriff's car pulls up next to a car with an old lady driving an old man. They are near a traffic light at Athen's Pizza on North Decatur. On the car's antenna, is a small, American flag. The lady stares at Brent and smiles.

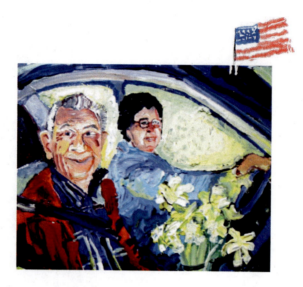

J"I. S'4fetfave'1 qt tl.e- Sbtte ment•J Hospih I
Safe Haven at the State Mental Hosp.

EXT. GEORGIA MENTAL HEALTH INSTITUTE   DAY

The police car pulls into the parking lot. The sun is bright. The acronym CIA comes to mind for the first time. The buildings of GMHI look big and ominous. The architecture is from the 1960's and 70's. From the outside, they look like experimental science buildings.

INT. GEORGIA MENTAL HEALTH INSTITUTE--------------DAY

Brent, still handcuffed, grins at his freedom from small architectural encasings. The handcuffs are released, and he is put in a locked unit with people that seem more lucid. The building has natural light. He is given a real meal. The floors no longer seem to be

These buildings later TV series, Stranger Things we.re,' useA to J"' {'he,

a trampoline. Brent is relieved there are female nurses on the unit. He feels safe and pampered, being able to use a private toilet.

INT. GEORGIA MENTAL HEALTH INSTITUTE\DR.S OFFICE\---------------DAY

> DR.
> Hello, Brent. My name is Dr. *(John Doe)*. How you doing?
>
> BRENT
> Fair-to-middling.
>
> DR.
> Do you know where you are?
>
> BRENT
> GMHT. My mom used to work in the psych unit, but I don't know which building.
>
> DR.
> Did you say your mom was a psych nurse here?
>
> BRENT
> Yes, in the forensics unit. But, I think, she now works at Regional on Panther's Ville Rd.
>
> DR.
> Oh, okay. Tell me a little about yourself.
>
> BRENT
> I'm an artist.
>
> DR.
> Oh, really. I'm into art a little. What kind of art do you do?

Brent starts rambling; he doesn't know where to start or end sentences. Nothing seems coherent.

> DR.
> So, what gallery did you say you were going to show at?

> BRENT
> At *(prestigious gallery)*. It's a pretty good gallery.

The doctor's eyes go still. He continues to take notes.

> DR.
> Well, let's see if we can find out what's wrong. Do you use any kind of recreational or illegal drugs?

> BRENT
> Everyone is asking that. I've only been around a few people who do them. I personally, have never had any.

> DR.
> At a cursory glance, from our records and what the police have said, it looks like you have had some kind of psychedelic. You sure you haven't been around any LSD?

> BRENT
> I have a vague memory of being at a friend's house, and they were talking about some kind of drug. I KNOW I turned down taking any.

> DR.
> What else do you remember?

> BRENT
> I had a beer... and a guy made some weird comment about it.

> DR.
> Any idea how long ago that was?

> BRENT
> No. I think it was awhile before all this happened.

> DR.
> Can you guess at how long?

> BRENT
> Maybe a week before I went to jail, but I don't know.

>   DR.
>   LSD can do some strange things. The question is how long it would
>   have stayed in your system. Do you know how long you were
>   incarcerated?
>
>   BRENT
>   No.

Doctor continues with his notes.

>   DR.
>   We cannot rule out an illness, but I'm guessing right now, it is drug
>   related. Your parents are asking for a blood test. Do you mind signing
>   this so we can draw some blood for them? We would like to draw
>   some, too.
>
>   BRENT
>   No problem. Why do Mom and Dad want to do that?
>
>   DR.
>   They want to check to see if any toxins from your paints could have
>   caused all this. Their blood tests will actually be more extensive than
>   ours. They say this is really out of character for you. After a few
>   more questions, you can get cleaned up.

INT. GMHI SHOWER ----------DAY

Brent revels in the personal shower. He can not remember the last one he had. Then, he remembers the string on his finger. It is wet for the first time, and he realizes the string won't last forever.

A MENTAL HEALTH EMPLOYEE pokes his head into the bathroom.

>   MENTAL HEALTH EMPLOYEE
>   Hey! Brent? Are you okay in there?
>
>   BRENT
>   I am OKAY! How big is your hot water heater?
>
>   MENTAL HEALTH EMPLOYEE
>   You've got another hour, if you want it.

This is where the original version of This story ended... Not now...

Haldol.

> BRENT
> Side effects?

> BRENT
> I'll take it!

INT. GMHI NURSE'S WINDOW------------DAY

Brent is called to the desk. A nurse explains that he will need some medication.

> BRENT
> What did you say this stuff was? And they do what?

> NURSE
> One is called Haldol, and the other is Cogentin. Haldol will help you relax a little and let your mind settle. You will feel more like yourself. The other, Cogentin, is to prevent side effects of the

> NURSE
> The Haldol can cause several, but we don't want you to get tardive dyskinesia.

> BRENT
> I don't even know what that is.

> NURSE
> Basically, it is uncontrolled movements in the face and tongue. It usually happens when people are on medicines like Haldol for a long time, especially without other meds to prevent it. You see it more in the older generation of patients. Do you see the older man over there with the tongue movements? But do not worry, you are not going to be on these very long.

> BRENT
> What's your name?

> NURSE
> (Jane)

Haldol + Cogentin =

> BRENT
> Why do you wear your badges turned around?

No answer.

> BRENT
> *Jane,* would you take these if you were me?

> NURSE (smiling)
> I cannot answer that question.

> BRENT (taking the pills)
> I am trusting you. By the way, it's nice to see women on the unit.

> NURSE
> It won't be long before you start feeling better.

INT. BRENT'S ROOM GMHI ---------DAY

Brent wants out. He keeps looking at the windows.

> BRENT (VO.)
> If I break another window and try to escape, I won't get far. could possibly go to the Greenhouse. I used to live there, and it's only two blocks away. The police would find me, and I have no money. That is just not a good idea.

Brent's new roommates are a Hindu from India, and a man with a beard and a Bible. There are approximately six bunks in the room, but only Brent and his two roommates.

Brent introduces himself to MR. HINDU, but all the man wants to talk about is the oneness of the universe.

> MR. HINDU
> There is no personal Cod.

> BIBLE MAN (to Brent)
> Do you believe in Jesus?

Brent's brain is *really* slow, now. He wants to converse, but can't keep up.

Cloudy, lethargy, Fog, Slowness

> BRENT
> I- I- I- UMM - Yes.

> BIBLE MAN
> You are a Christian?

Brent stares at Bible Man.

> BRENT
> Yes.

> BIBLE MAN
> Well, it says right here...

BIBLE MAN opens his big Bible.

> BIBLE MAN
> ...that unless you cut your hair, you are going to hell.

Brent slumps.

> BRENT
> I - I - don't think that's what it means. *(long pause)* Didn't Jesus have long hair?

Brent's eyelids are hanging low.

> BIBLE MAN
> It IS pretty clear. Cross reference it with this verse, right here.

> BRENT
> I think I want to watch TV.

> BIBLEMAN
> God is going to speak to you to repent.

Brent sits to watch TV, but is not interested in *Jeopardy*. Brent explores the building.

INT. WALK IN GMHI BUILDING   DAY

Brent goes to the opposite side of th e buildin g and passes a room with a small w ind ow. He loo ks in. It is Pep to Bis mol pink, but a tad da rker. In the middl e o f the room is a lone table with strap s. The room is very menacin g.

> BR ENT (V O.)
> Peter? *(pause)* God, where am I? I fee l lik e a rat in a maze. At least there are "scientists" here, and they seem mor e personabl e. Peter, are these your scientists?

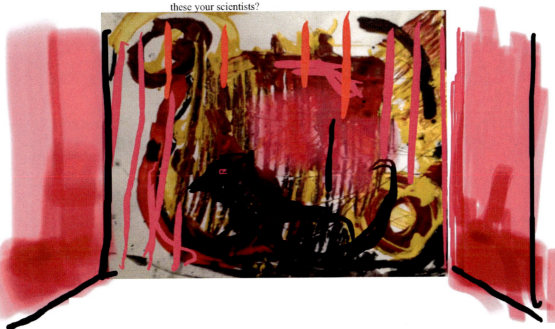

No res pon se from any voices.

> BRENT (V O.)
> God, I don't know what voice in my head to trust. God is silent. Peter is gone? What is MY mind ? I'm having a hard time distinguishing my thoughts and God 's direct ion... and whatever the hell else is affe ctin g m e.

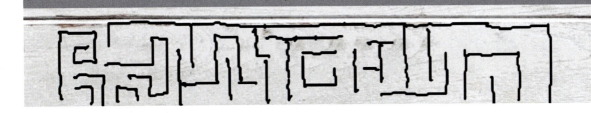

Brent walks to the open lobby adjacent to the strap room. Brent looks down at the journal in his hand. On the cover is a sketch of a lighthouse. It reads "60 lb. Medium Weight Drawing Paper."

          BRENT (VO.)
          Where did THIS come from? I'm surprised they have left me with a spiral, metal-bounded sketchbook?

Brent looks down at a man on the floor sleeping on a mat.

          BRENT
          What are you doing over here?

          MANON MAT
          I'm on suicide watch. They say they can see me better over here.

          BRENT
          Why are you depressed?

          MANON MAT
          I just am. Lost my job. Lost all my money. Lost my wife...

As he is listening, Brent looks up. There, above the man on the mat, is a mural on the wall. It is a painting of a beach and sailboats. The colors do not register in Brent's mind. Brent smiles and sits down.

          BRENT (VO.)
          At least the waves are not YELLOW!

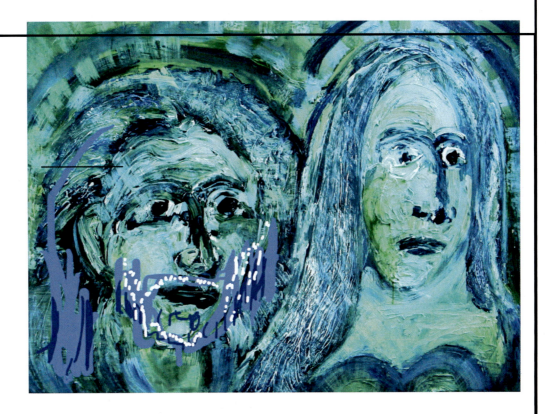

He looks at the restroom door. Brent pulls out his pen and sketches the beach mural on the first page of his journal. He uses a blue pen like his sketch at Corfu. He continues talking with the man.

        BRENT
        What do you think of that painting?

        MANonMAT
        Takes money to go there. I'll never see it again... and no woman wants
        a man without money... at my age.

        BRENT
        Despair is real, isn't it?

Brent tells him about the time he was at **L' Abri**. The man does not seem interested. They sit in quiet.

INT. GMHI WITH T ----------DAY

As he nears the end of the drawing, Brent gets a call from the nurse's station. *T*, one of Brent's pastors from the PCA church, comes WHISTLING around the corner.

> BRENT
> Hey, *T!* How did you get in here?
>
> T. *(smiling)*
> I walked through that wall over there... using the DOOR.
> Actually, pastors have certain inalienable rights. I can get in here, but your parents will not be able to. They send a hug.

They walk to TV lobby. Brent is mentally far behind *T*.

> T.
> Heard you took a trip up the mountain! *(smiling)* And busted
> into the radio tower... through the WINDOW? Did you by chance come
> down with some STONE tablets from the Mountain? Just kidding!!!

Brent actually has a good laugh and proceeds to break down and starts telling This story and love for *E*.

> BRENT
> I heard your whistle in Grant Park. You wanted me to follow you
> so I could show up at the wedding with *E*.

T looks a little stunned.

> T
> That wasn't me! What you are telling me doesn't make sense. Brent,
> what you are telling me isn't real. It is not truth. But, I love you anyway.

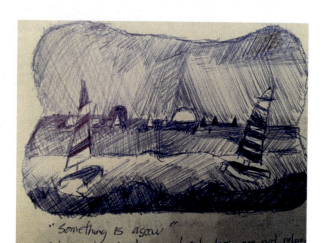

"Something is ascew"

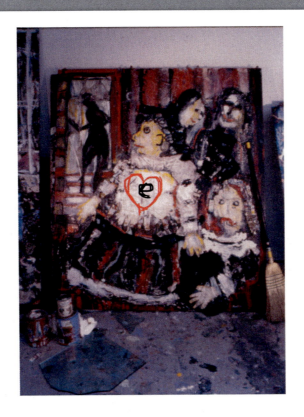
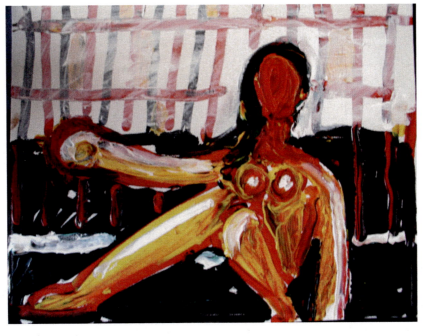

ep

INT. GMHI TV LOBBY ROOM WITH 'T' ---------DAY

Braves baseball comes on over the TV. It's a much better TV than the one in jail cell ElA. Brent stares at the TV as Smoltz, a pitcher, gets a hit. *T* watches baseball with Brent for a long while. Not much is said, as Brent checks out mentally and writes a poem.

        T.
        Didn't know you write?

        BRENT
        Most of it doesn't make sense when **T** go back and read it.

        T.
        Do you mind sharing what you wrote?

Brent shows This beach drawing and the poem **in** his sketchbook. BRENT

WRITES:

"God still gives meaning to the abyss of baseball. Stats, mats, and hats,... and bats, ...and chats. Christ heals the hits, the pits, and the mits."

        T.
        Not bad, for a painter. Do you want to talk about the poem?

        BRENT
        Not really. I'm getting tired.

        T.
        Okay.. Ts there anythin g T can br i ng to you on my next visit?

        BRENT
        There is a tremend ous screened in porch over there where the smokers hang ou t. I don't smoke cigarettes, but the screened in porch is the closest place I can go to get to the outside.

r s+a/lJ2..,
Sac/4 ,·n r air.
Tr ec¾ry'   I had no idea

2 decades lost

But He's the Boss.

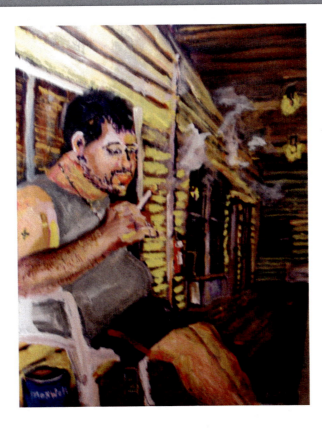

Brent tears up.

BRENT
It's the only place I can smell the rain.

[Pause]

BRENT
I can only take the smell of these cleaners around here for so long. Could you bring me a cigar?

T just stares at Brent, then smiles.

T. (loudly)
A Ciiiiiigar!!! *(pause)* Sure, what kind? What's your favorite brand?

> BRENT
> It really doesn't matter. You know, my first cigar, I skipped a physics test that I knew I was going to fail. I sat out back of the testing auditorium and inhaled the whole thing. I was by myself and didn't know not to inhale. My lungs burned for days.

T and Brent hug. It is the first physical contact he has had in a week. Brent remembers something and goes to his room. He gets a white bag and hands it to T. Inside is his jail outfit.

> BRENT
> T, I almost forgot, will you give this to my parents for me? T'd like it as a souvenir and reminder for the days to come.

> T. (jokingly)
> Before you climb the mountain again, give me a call!

T leaves with bag in hand.
[Scene pans to Brent smoking a cigar with the smokers on the porch. It is raining.]

> SMOKER
> Where did he get that? Haven't seen one like that in a long time!

INT. BRENT'S ROOM GMHI ---------DAY

Brent dreams that his parents are just outside the main entrance. The nurse lets them into the foyer between the unit's locked doors and the building's outside doors. By law, Brent cannot see them. Brent is briefly let into the "in-between" space and sees his parents for the first time. The family is technically not on the unit, and Brent is still in the building. He dreams that their car drives by the porch on a cloudy, overcast day. The rain falls. He knows they are praying for him. He also dreams of conversations with his parents, grandmother, and sistet; on the phone.

INT. DR #2'S OFFICE (GMHII ---------DAY

Brent gets a new doctor.

Grey is for memory of Stone Mountain

DR. #2
Hi, Brent. I'm Dr. *(X)*. By the records, it looks like you are doing a little better. The Haldol and Cogentin must be doing their job. How do you feel?

BRENT
I'm very confused about what is happening, but I want to thank you for having better food here.

DR. #2 *(laughing)*
Yeah, they bring the food in from a pretty good cafeteria for the men here. How is your mood?

BRENT
I feel okay. My brain seems to operate clearer, though I am confused about the past events.

DR. #2
No homicidal or suicidal thoughts of any kind?

BRENT
No.

DR. #2
We have run the blood tests. Nothing out of the ordinary. We tested you for everything! Apparently, your parents wanted to know all possibilities of cause. It's good, and not so good, news. There is no probable drug cause, outside of a drug we are not aware of. There are always new "designer drugs," but I don't think this is the cause. You were under a lot of financial stress and not sleeping, right?

BRENT
Yes.

DR. #2
It is possible you just had a temporary break of some kind. And, it is possible that you may have some mental disorder. Unfortunately, it is not my job to make that diagnosis at this moment. It is basically my job to get you clear enough to get you out of here.

> BRENT
> Where am I going to go next?

> DR. #2
> Unfortunately, that's up to the law. You will probably be back in incarceration until either a bond is posted, or until a court trial.

Brent slumps in his chair, feeling an abandonment.

> DR. #2
> Personally, I think it won't be long, and if you need treatment, you may get it better outside of these walls.

> BRENT
> By the way, what happened to my last doctor? It may be good for him to see my improvement.

> DR. #2 *(clears his throat)*
> He needed to drop your case for personal reasons.

> BRENT
> What?

> DR. #2 *(staring straight at Brent)*
> Let's just say his wife runs a "particular" gallery in town.

> BRENT
> You're kidding me!

> DR. #2 *(still staring straight at Brent)*
> You're going to be okay. You seem like a good kid. Just what were you doing up on the mountain, anyway? *(pause)* Actually, I do not need to know.

Brent just stares back at the doctor.

> BRENT
> You really want to know? It is a convoluted love story.

DR. #2
It's okay, Brent. It was good to meet you. Good luck, and do NOT hesitate to get help if things get rough later. There ARE ways to get help.

(Chess at E!A)

INT. ORANGE JAIL COMMON ROOM E1A ···•··· DAY

Brent sits calmly, playing chess with a roommate in the common room. El A is not the raging machine it once was. [The window has been replaced in the door with STRONG PLEXI.] Brent sees two men; they are looking at him and subtly pointing.

CELLMATE 1
Rumors say he's the one who got past the shadow.

CELLMATE 2
It has not been done. It's NOT meant to be possible.

CELLMATE 1
He's changed the game!

CELLMATE 2
If so, you know how high up that is?

CELLMATE 1
That's well beyond the Special Forces.

CELLMATE 2
How did he fight?

CELLMATE 1
Don't know.

CELLMATE 2
Get up there to that level, and no telling who he was talking to.

CELLMATE 1
Don't you remember? We all could tell something was up that night. Daniel in the Den! We felt it down here.

They shake their heads. Brent intensely stares back at them, but is really just curious what they know about the shadow. He never asks, though.

CHESS BUDDY
I see you got your mind back.

BRENT
What do you mean?

CHESS BUDDY
Before, when you were here, you would mostly play with the pieces off the board. You were elsewhere. When you finally tried to focus, I beat you in several moves. You didn't really even remember the moves. Now, there is no way I can win at this game against you.

BRENT
I have played hundreds of chess games, but I'm really not that good.

CHESS BUDDY
Look around. Boredom is a huge problem in here. See that white guy? He sleeps all the time. No purpose. It's BAD! See him?

CHESS BUDDY points to the man who just sits on the edge of his bed, staring.

BRENT
Why does he never move?

CHESS BUDDY
It's like he is in some kind of shock, or something.

BRENT
Before, I got the strange sense that underneath the stiff facade, he is a decent human being.

CHESS BUDDY
I've seen him get nasty, but only rarely.

BRENT
He never was to me. He just sat there on his bed pointing in the same pose. He looked like a chess piece himself, a Knight.

CHESS BUDDY
When are you gettin' out of here?

BRENT
Don't know, at least a couple days.

CHESS BUDDY
You should know that between 2-3, you can go to the gym. And, for about 15 minutes, they will let you stand outside in the yard.

BRENT
I don't remember any of that. Before, I did see a long blade of grass on the floor and thought someone put it there as a form of witchcraft, or something.

CHESS BUDDY
Someone probably did bring it in and put it on the floor. Maybe just as a reminder of the outside. You have probably realized that the small things become huge, in the crib.

BRENT
Yeah, the immediacy of present awareness and proximity.

CHESS BUDDY
You're definitely not from around here.

BRENT
What time did you say the gym opens?

A guard opens the door to El A, the one with the window that Brent busted.

GUARD
Time for meds.

BRENT (looking at CHESS BUDDY)
I don't remember that last time.

CHESS BUDDY
Some of these people do better on pills.

BRENT
But I don't remember them giving pills out last time, and I was here for awhile.

> CHESS BUDDY (*with a crazy look on his face*)
> Maybe it was in the food.

The guard starts yelling out names. Brent does not hear his name and walks up to the guard slowly.

> BRENT
> Hey, I've recently been on meds at GMHI. I think I'm suppose to have them.

> GUARD
> Your name is not on the list. It would probably take at least a couple days before the proper paper work gets here from GMHI.

> BRENT
> I think I need them.

> GUARD
> You're S-O-L until I get the proper paperwork.

Brent later goes to the gym by himself. He shoots a few basketball hoops. He returns to E1A, and through a small window in an empty side cell, watches a storm roll in. He is mesmerized by the purple and blue bruise like colors against the orange wall. He sleeps in 15 minute intervals, for what seems to be days.

INT. JAIL GYM (CHURCH SERVICE)------------DAY

GUARD comes to the door.

> GUARD
> Those with an green wrist band can go to the church service in the gym.

Brent looks at his wrist band and heads out in line. He thinks about his wrist band and questions its color. He thinks it once was orange. Inmates from all over the jail are sitting on the floor in the gym. Brent is aware he is one of the few white guys surrounded by a hundred people. The white preacher walks in and talks about "Hope."

> PREACHER
> "...When you get out of here, you will need a job. The Bible says to work, to give unto Caesar what is Caesar's. Here are

some ways to start your own business. You will need a business license... the proper tax forms..."

The preacher then gives a long listed column of instructions. Nobody is taking notes. Brent lean over to an acquaintance from ElA.

> BRENT
> You gotta be kidding me. Is this for real? He is talking so far above the needs of people in here, it's not even funny. Some of these people have totally lost their mind, and those who haven't, probably will not remember his twelve steps after they leave here.

None-the-less, Brent goes up and talks to the preacher afterwards. The preacher hands Brent a tract and starts to ask questions. When Brent has answered them sufficiently, he tries to recruit Brent to lead a Bible study in ElA. Brent walks away, wanting nothing to do with it. As Brent is lead back to ElA, a JAIL MATE with dreads approaches.

> JAIL MATE
> Do you know where I can get some dope around here?

Brent looks at him kind of funny 'cause it was at the end of a "church" service.

> BRENT
> Sorry, I don't do drugs.

Jail mate looks at Brent's ElA wrist band, and snickers.

> JAIL MATE
> Oh? You are one of those. From the land of pills. You got any of those instead?

> BRENT
> No.

> JAIL MATE (in a derogatory manner)
> What ya doing in here?

> BRENT
> I busted out some windows. A couple on Stone Mountain, and a big one at the Courthouse across the street. Then, I got ElA.

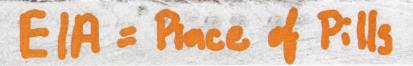

                    JAIL MATE (smiling)
                Now, that's what I am talking about! I didn't think you were
                THAT guy.

Brent smiles.

                    JAIL MATE (yelling to his friends)
                YO!!! Shit! This is the guy who smashed in the Courthouse
                window!

Brent watches inmates come toward him.

                    JAIL MATE (looking at Brent)
                Why did you do it? What's the connection between Stone Mountain
                and the Courthouse?

                    BRENT
                Not sure, now.

                    JAIL MATE
                NOT sure?

Brent heads back to E1A before he is the center of attention.

INT. ORANGE COMMON ROOM E1A ------------DAY

Brent, back in E1A, lies on his bed thinking for an undistinguishable amount of time.

                    BRENT (V.O.)
                T says what I went through was not real. You there, Peter?

No response. Brent looks at his finger; the string is still there.

                    BRENT (V.O.)
                Something sure as hell happened to me. It was not all a dream. No
                telling what those GMHI meds did to me.

EXT. POND - HILL AT EMORY UNIV. ----- EVENING----------------FLASHBACK

Brent, £, and Mike are rolling down the hill near the pond, racing to the bottom. There is much laughter in the dizziness of the moment. Brent, later at dark, is sitting on a rock with £, next to the pond. He puffs, but not inhales, on the first cigarette that has ever touched his lips.

INT. EXIT ORANGE COMMON ROOM E1A ----- DAY

>BRENT (V.O.)
>They have let me keep the string on through the processing at GMHI and back into jail.

Guard opens door to E1A.

>GUARD
>Brent Weston, gather your stuff.

Brent laughs a little to himself, looking at a bed that only has a sheet and roll of toilet paper.

>BRENT (VO.)
>Are they going to reuse my toilet paper? Surely not .. Just give it to another inmate.

>CELLMATE3
>Remember, my name is *(Joe Smith)!* Maybe your lawyer can get me out, too.

>CELLMATE4
>Another one bites the dust.

>CELLMATE5
>He ain't coming back. Free bird! That bird is FREEEEE!

>CELLMATE 6
>No telling where he is going.

>CELLMATE5
>No telling where that Mo' Fo' has been.

CELLMATE 1
See ya, shadow buster.

Brent bows his head and looks back at a relatively calm room. Several men are just staring with a sad smile, except for one man who is yelling.

CELLMATE3
IT'S NOT FAIR. IT'S NOT FAIR. His family must have money for a lawyer. He comes from one of those rich families.

CELLMATE5
Remember us!

1,. Tripp,,., w.-u. +a-e. 1'ople of ~~AirplQnes~~

INT. WHITE CELL of former BAT SCENE -------------DAY

Brent look s at the window in the door as he leaves El A. He is escorted to the WHITE CELL where he saw the bat shadow.

BRENT (to the sheriff)
Could you tell me what is behind that door over there with the shadow?

The sheriff stops and looks directly at Brent.

SHERIFF
Mops. Nothing but MOPS! For WASHING the floors. Got it?

The door is locked behind Brent. Brent instantly hears something coming throu gh the wall. H e goes to the left wall and puts his ear up to it. With his hand , he draws a circle on the wall and punctuates the middle with a thud. Surprisingly, he hears a thud back. He tries it again and backs away from the wall, quickly. He barely hears the thud this time. This sound is not only in his head. He starts to calculate the sound. The distance from the wall makes a difference in *his* calculations. He now knows someone is in the cell next to him. Then he puts his ear to the wall and hears the song "I'll Fly Away, Oh Glory." It sounds like a small church service in the next room over. Brent remember s the fly that once entered the cell to be with him.

PETER (VO.)
Brent. Brent. *(pause)* Brent.

230

Brent immediately stops and looks around. He gets up and goes to the wall where the song was coming from.

> PETER (VO.)
> You are making us laugh, Brent. Check the wall all you want, and mea8ure your di8tance8.

Brent immediately hears the difference in sounds. This one is not coming from the wall. This one seems omnidirectional. This has bypassed normal hearing. He notices when he raises an arm, the ear on that side has a tone.

> BRENT (V O.)
> Shit. Great. You again. Where have you been? Y'all left me hanging.

> PETER (VO.)
> Actually, the contrary.

> BRENT
> What do you mean?

> PETER (VO.)
> We have been here the whole time. First, some of my colleagues want to apologize for putting you through the cell near the hooded people.

> BRENT
> Y'all put me through hell, you fuckers.

> PETER (VO.)
> Brent, no need for the language, but we understand! Ever thought about how abandoned Christ felt on the cross?

[Long silence]

> PETER (VO.)
> Those hooded people were real, but the woman doing yoga... Brent, your mind was scrambled almost to the death. Do you remember those geometric patterns you analyzed in your mind?

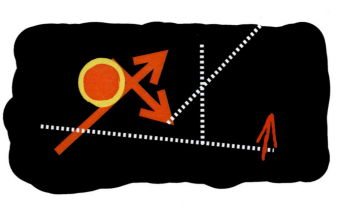

BRENT(VO.)
I'm beginning to remem ber. Some of them were bea u tiful, and some of the m were horr ific. The bad ones repea ted after certain types of thoughts. They were going very fast, and I was having an emo tion al response to each one. How did you get those into my head with my eyes closed?

PETER (VO)
Chinese secret... First inni ng and you have already struck out. THINK it, don't say it.

BRENT
What?

[Pause]

BRENT (V.O.)
Oh, baseball! *(pause)* By the way, how are the Brav es doin g ?

PETER (VO.)
Let me check. *(pause)* Rock solid.

BRENT(V.O.)
Stone Mountain?

BRENT
Funny.

PETER (V.O.
Smolt zee is hav ing a great year.

BRE NT (V.O.)
Their pitching is really good.

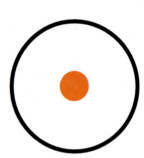

PETER (VO.)
Apparently, so is your s! You hit the bull's eye with the orange... On that wall. You were really angry, yet still agile. No jud gm ent on my part. Considering what you were going through, you needed that release .

Brent starts to see images flash behind his eye lids again.

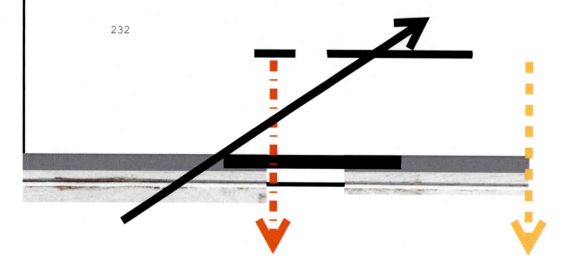

BRENT (VO.)
Haven't we bee n thr ou gh thi s befo re?

PETER (VO.)
Chinese secret?

BRENT (VO.)
Whatever you wan t to call it.

PETER (VO.)
T w ant you to li e b ack on the floo r and rel ax w it h your eyes closed.

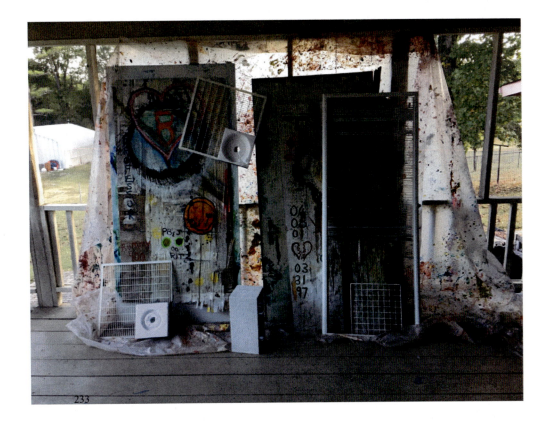

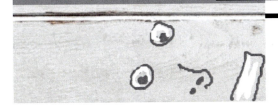

Brent lies down on the floor. Instead of seeing static images that change every few seconds, they begin to morph. He tries to focus by pushing blood into his eyes at various pressures. Soon, he is seeing line drawings of aircraft flying through the sky. Planes, highly detailed in their movements and precision, are darting across the gray background in his mind.

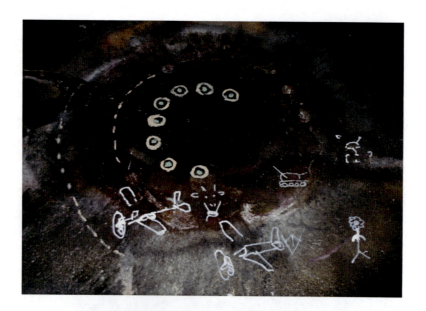

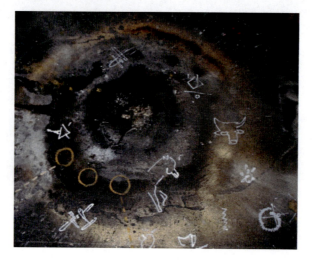

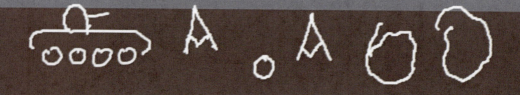

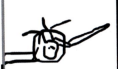 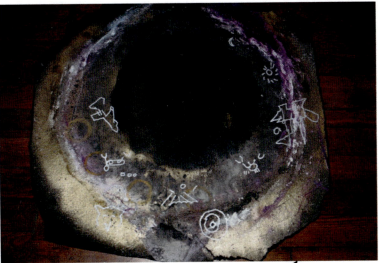 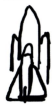

BRENT (VO.)

PETER (V O.)

Old plane, but you just hit a homerun!

BRENT (VO.)
Ahhh, umm, tha t's pretty impressive.

PETER (VO.)
Tell me what colors you are seeing.

BRENT (v.0.)
Basica lly, various types of gray with moving lines.

PETER (VO .)
Brent, do you know that people like me may never get to experience wha t you just saw?

Brent's audible mind goes quiet.

BRENT (VO.)
I wish I could see where you work. It would be nice to meet you in PERSON!

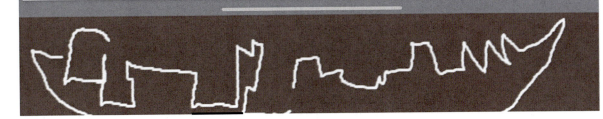

PETER (VO.)
Not going to happen ! But you will be trained to wa tch for us.

BRENT (VO.)
If YOUR training and experimentin g proceeds like it has been, there may be nothing of me remaining.

PETER (VO.)
Trust in our God and in US. See if you can tell me what we are puttin g on our screen now.

Brent's body is barely mov in g, but his tempe rature is okay. Soon, Brent begins to see some lime green lines star t to form in his head. He waits as they untan gle themselves into a scientific drawing of a gird ed space shuttle. The shuttle starts to rotate without moving across his mind . The grid stays in full perspective from each angle, and then it vanishes like the lights were turned out.

BRENT (V.O .)
That's...

PETER (VO) (interrupting)
What?

BRENT (VO.)
...was a space sh uttle.

PETER (VO.)
Two for two .

BRENT (VO.)
The lines were in greenish color?

PETER (VO.)
You bea t me to the question.

BRENT
Don't tell me you can do this in color. Can you pro je ct a color movie into the mind?

PETER (V O.)
The answer is no, not with the clarity you are thinking about . It IS si mply ama zin g that you can see what you did. You are about

85 % on the cusp of what we can do. We will try and run some full color after a few more tests. Hold on a minute. 1 actually have to go to the restroom myself. 1 will be back shortly. How are you doing?

BRENT (V O.)
Okay, but take me *to* the deep waters of Corfu sometime ?

No response as Brent is questioning his puzzled mind.

FRIENDLY WOMAN (VO.)
Hey, Brent. My name is C h ris. J ha ve the COMM until Pete gets back. I fina lly get my turn in the lead, but only shortly.

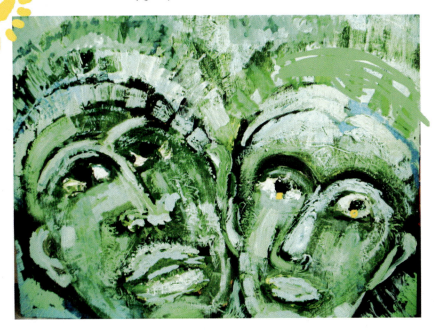

BRENT (VO.)

Bridge to Stone Arena

Hi, Chris. How did you get here?

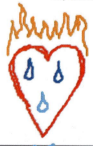
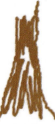

CHRTS (V.O.)
How does anyone get anywhere? I can say there was a lot of studying, at least a year on your case alone.

BRENT
Bullshit?

CHRIS (V.O.)
"Bullshit?" Way to meet a stranger!

BRENT (V.O.)
Sorry, your voice sounds quite friendly. Mind me asking how old you are?

CHRIS (V.O.)
I'm about your age, believe it or not.

BRENT (V.O.)
Please, tell me you are single.

CHRIS (V.O.)
Actually, divorced.

BRENT (V.O.)
Sorry to hear that, but I do feel relieved.

CHRIS (V.O.)
Appreciate the empathy, but back to a quick comment or two.

BRENT (V.O.)
I ain't got nowhere to go.

CHRIS (V.O.)
I'm not kidding, I have been assigned to your case. And Lord willing, will be for the long haul.

BRENT (V.O.)
Chris, do your best to take care of me.

CHRIS (V.O.)
God has gotten me here, AND I have earned it. Brent, you are a remarkable person. God has also been with you.

BRENT (V.O.)
Yeah, but I haven't earned it. Sounds like you are a Christian.

CHRIS (V.O.)
I am.

BRENT (V.O.) (smiling)
You're not going to make me cut my hair to remain "saved," are you?

CHRIS (V.O.)
Are you thinking about BIBLE MAN?

BRENT
Can't y'all read my mind?

CHRIS (V.O.)
The system is not foolproof, Brent. Got it? And it's BIBLE MAN, isn't it?

BRENT (V.O.)
Yes.

CHRIS (V.O.)
God loves that man, too! His plight could have been yours. And besides, I am not his judge, nor yours.

BRENT (V.O.)
You know what my plight is now? I can not seem to trust the Holy Spirit talking to me. I am beginning to think that if this technology is used on a grand scale, many Christians could be deceived, and I'm not even bringing up any privacy of mind issues.

CHRIS (V.O.)
Slooooooow down, hold your horses. Not currently possible the way you are envisioning it, and theoretically...

BRENT (VO.) *(interrupting)*

...and theoretically, if I am one of the few in the know of this technology, I may just fall into a superiority complex.

CHRIS (V O.)

Brent, our leaders and scientists have to deal with the superiority issues, as well. After all, what do you think fueled Hitler's projects? A superiority mindset. It is important to note though, that some of our scientists originally came from Germany, during and after the war. These scientists' work and LIVES are now being redeemed. America is the great melting pot and the
"shining city on a hill." This is serious. I appreciate your concern on the subject.

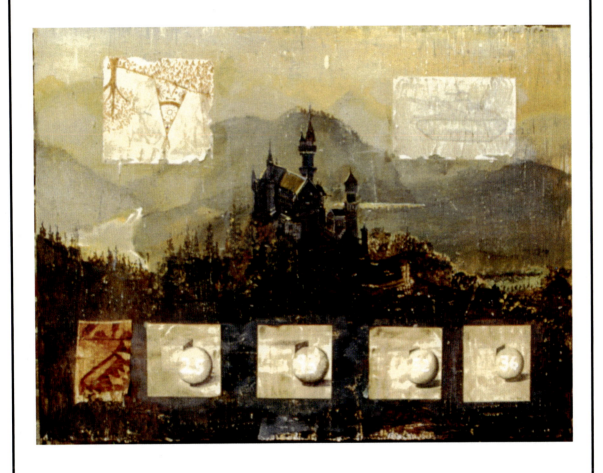

BRENT *(long pause)*
Oh, God.

CHRIS *(V O.)*
Don't worry about all this right now, or the superiority issues. So far, you have been able to drop them. Hi, Pete! Everything come out okay?

PETER *(VO.)*
Funny. So, how is it going Chris?

BRENT *(VO.)* *(to himself)*
How am I going to explain this to Mom and Dad?

CHRIS *(V O.)*
A little tes ty, but we have met.

PETER *(V.O.)*
Nothing says you have to tell your parents, but Chris will be here to help.

BRENT *(VO.)*
Are you cute?

CHRIS *(V O.)* *(quickly)*
Average! Brent, I will be here awhile yet tonight, but it's time for me to relinquish center stage. "May we live long and prosper."

BRENT *(V.O .)*
"May the force be with us."

PETER *(V.O.)*
That's the ticket.

BRENT *(V O.)*
Good to meet you, Chris!

CHRIS *(VO.)*
You too, Brent.

> PETER (VO.)
> Back to work. Those airplanes. Brent we are going to have them moving with your eyes shut, and when we say so, we want you to slowly open your eyes. That's it, got it.

Brent is lying on the floor. He occasionally opens his eyes.

> BRENT (VO.)
> The afterimage lasts between 1 and 10 seconds, depending on the original image.

> PETER (VO.)
> Okay, now we want you to keep your eyes open.

Brent sees outlines of planes very faintly.

> BRENT (V.O.)
> I can barely see the planes.

> PETER (VO.)
> That is okay. Now, be as still as you can with eyes shut.

> BRENT (V O.)
> I don't see much. I don't see "Da plaaan e... Da plaaane."

A minute or two goes by. Brent sees an abstract painting in colors start to morph. They start spinning in perfect geometries. For a few seconds, he sees a glowing kaleidoscope. Then in an instant, lights out. There is a temporary afterglow.

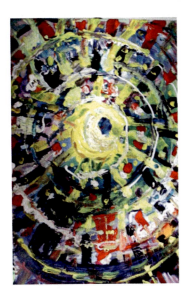

BRENT (VO.)
Now, that looked like what I would expect from LSD, or something.

PETE (VO.) (kind of laughing)
Brent, we got you up to about 93% of what we can do. This is very rare. A little room for improvement, but give us time.

BRENT (VO.)
Well, I seem to have A LOT of that these days.

PETER (VO.)
A lot of what?

BRENT (VO.)
Time!

PETER (V.O.)
You will be out of here before you know it.

Without hesitation.

PETER (VO.)
Brent, technology will soon be better with the definition of color. The best way to describe the kaleidoscope is a "combo." The gray lines were mixed with colors as much as we could control them. If you're curious, the grey line technology has been around longer
than you might think. Color is being refined as we speak. We had a breakthrough with it a couple years back.

BRENT (V.O.)
With this stuff, I bet you can affect dreams.

PETER (VO.)
The answer to that is yes, and no. There is still an extensive amount of research that has to go into dreams, how to understand and influence them.

BRENT (VO.) (to himself)
This is crazy. I already have issues with my dreams in here. I don't know what was dream and what was not.

PETER (V.O.)
To be expected!

BRENT (V.O.) (to himself)
Maybe it's possible for the mind to receive frequencies, but there is no way they can read it, especially without some kind of device near. There ain't one in this room; I can see that. It is also possible that thoughts could be "interjected" at such a rate that all voices themselves, including mine, are faster than regular thought. I could be "receiving" entire conversations. Basically, in a relaxed state, I'm just listening to "both" sides talk - "them" and "me." Possibly, the "me" is also a projection of the computer people.

PETER (VO.)
You are now beginning to think. That's a fairly interesting assumption Brent, but that is not how we normally work. Not to say that cannot be done, but it is a little more dangerous.

BRENT (V.O.)
Peter, basically you are "saying" that I am not just a very relaxed "receiver," but I am a "transmitter?"

PETER (VO.)
In the most basic scenario, isn't that true? You have your senses and a MOUTH!

9

BRENT
It ain't that easy!

PETER (VO.)
"He swings and misses."

BRENT (VO.)
How am I suppose to take the fact that I am a transmitter?

PETER (VO.)
It may not be that easy for you.

BRENT (VO.)
It's apparently not so easy for you and your computers, either. Let's hit the refresh button! My transition to this moment was not the smoothest.

244

• Years after typing this story - there was an article printed how a guy from MIT invented a machine to read minds by reading mouth muscles.

PETER (VO.)
That's a fair statement.

BRENT (VO.)
And if I can really even receive, what the hell is 139 x 9325? Why can't you pop the answer into my head at any time?

PETER (VO.)
Wow! Where did that come from? And you failed physics?

BRENT (VO.) *(smiling)*
Tha t's right. TWICE, T think!

PETER (VO..)
Well then, how do you expect to understand what we could tell you even if we wanted to? But we cannot with our "broken connections." Also, we have developed a protocol over the years, protocol derived from experiences like yours.

BRENT (V O.)
Cop out!

PETER (VO.)
Precisely. *(long pause)* Give me a sec...

BRENT
Like, I'm STUCK, if you haven't noticed.

PETER (V.O.)
Actually, T want you to give me 36 secs., as in count to 36 the best you can. And STARE out the window.

BRENT (VO.)
1, 2..., 10..., 20..., 30, 31, 32, 33, 34, 35, 36!

Just as Brent hits 36, a sheriff comes around the corner and pauses right by the window. He takes a mop out of a bucket and starts mopping.

PETER (VO.)
Get the point!?

BRENT
SHIT! Did you make that happen, or did you just predict it correctly with a remote sensor?

PETER (V.O.)
First of all, "SHIT," is not generally in my lexicon. SHHH - IT may be a proper response in this case. In the future, our dilemma is going to be deciding when and where to remind you of events like today. Judging how loud to "speak to you," or knowing how far
to go to get a response, may also be a challenge. In coming years, technology is going to get fast, as in "warp" speed.

BRENT (V.O.)
I follow.

PETER (V.O.)
Now, get some rest.

Brent is awakened, and he is being moved to the building with the Courthouse. He can barely keep his eyes open. He has been told he is on his way out.

BRENT (to guard)
How long is it going to be?

GUARD
I don't know. There is a bunch of paper work. It's going to be awhile.

17. Psyc"olosy of the DQrk Window

INT. JAIL EXIT ROOM #1------------DAY

~~Brent is ushered into a roo~~m with approximately 20 men. It is a very small room with no bathrooms. People are talking amongst themselves and to themselves. Alcohol stench is in the air. An older African American almost passes out on the bench in front of Brent.
Brent feels like a sardine in the can. Someone throws up in the sink. Brent does not think he will be in this cell very long.

OP - ☐ IJ ☐ D

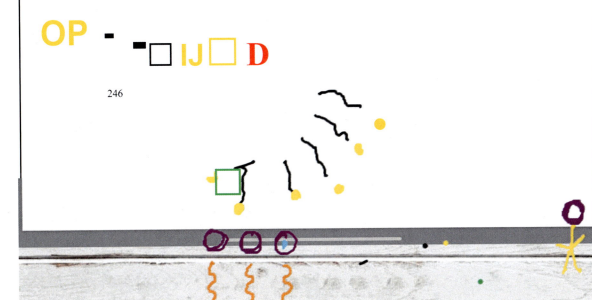

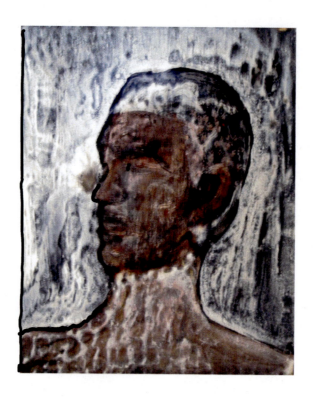

BRENT (VO.)
You there, Peter?

PETER (VO.)
We gotcha. What would you like to talk about?

BRENT (VO.)
Not sure! But I'd like to be out of here .

PETER (VO.)
Kick back, it's a crowded beach.

BRENT (V.O.)
I saw they fixed the window to the Courthouse.

PETER (VO.)
Of course. They had to fix that pretty quickly, and besides, that's in the past. The window is as good as new, just a percentage of a penny that is being spent on you. Brent, this is as good a
time as any to...

BRENT (VO.)
Ahhh! Here it comes!

PETER (VO.)
Since you brought up the window, let's talk about the WINDOWS, as in plural. You mind if Chris joins in? You and she ARE going to be a team for awhile.

BRENT (VO.)
No problem! Hey Chris.

CHRIS (V.O.)
Hey Brent. Good to be back. How are you doing?

BRENT (V O.)
Getting hungry, and I think they forgot to give me my lunch sack today in all the transitions. What did YOU have for breakfast? Must have been BEITER than mine.

CHRIS (V O.)
Yogurt, granola, and coffee.

PETER (V.O.) (to Brent)
You did not ask me that?

BRENT (V.O.)
You had me flying airplanes, remember.

PETER (V O.)
"But of course."

BRENT (VO.)
Dijon! You've been there, too? That was where I cried over my first painting.

248

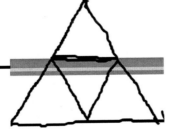

> PETER (VO.) *(talking to himself)*
> Me, too.

Brent is confused.

> CHRIS (VO.) *(to Pete, as 1/ Brent was not in the territory, but loud enough that Brent gets the hint)*
> Pete, you wanted to talk about the windows?

> PETER (VO.)
> Ah, yeeees, the wiiiiindows.

> BRENT (V O.) *(feeling a little ashamed)*
> I don't remember really breaking them out of anger. I had some kind of logic that seemed right at the time. And besides, I took the first window apart; it was already broken.

> PETER (V.O.) *(seriously)*
> BRENT. BRENT. BRENT!
> Rest in peace.
> *(then laughing a little)*
> And let the windows rest in PIECES!

> BRENT (VO.)
> Not funny!

Chris laughs in the background.

> PETER (V.O.)
> We want you to forget those windows for now.

> CHRIS (V O.)
> Brent, we know you had Psychology 101.

> BRENT (V O.)
> I don't remember a thing, except that my GA TECH psychology teacher had been a missionary to the Native Americans out West. But that is fuzzy. In the Architecture Department that seemed dedicated to the worldviews of Postmodernism, it was refreshing to meet staff who actually believed in an ultimate Creator that formed us with or without, evolution.

PETER (VO.)
We figured you wouldn't remember too much. Your memory skills are not bad, but neither are they the best. Book knowledge apparently, is not your thing. However, we have taken interest in a couple memories that you began to explore in Painting I at
GA State.

BRENT (VO.)
That was one of my favorite classes ever, if not THE fav!

CHRTS (V O.)
Tell us about your encaustic painting.

BRENT (VO.)
Oh, God. You mean the one about the garage door window?

PETER (V.O.)
You do remember the events?

BRENT (V O.)
Yes, but I don't know how accurate the memories are.

CHRIS (V O.)
That's okay. Let's just hash it out a bit. Whatever comes to mind, Brent, we are not making any judgments on you as a person here.

BRENT (VO.)
I cannot hide my thoughts anyway, can I?

PETER (VO.)
Very good question; hang onto that thought for another time. But for now, tell us about the painting.

BRENT (V O.)
I don't remember the assignment, but I ended up going back to the house I grew up in on Burlington Road to face a childhood memory. I took my easel and introduced myself to the guys that lived in the house, then. I told them I had grown up in the house as a kid, and I asked them if I could paint in the driveway. They said, "Yes, that would be fine."

CHRIS (V.O.)
You are doing well.

PETER (V.O.)
You must have been near the pine tree your parents planted?

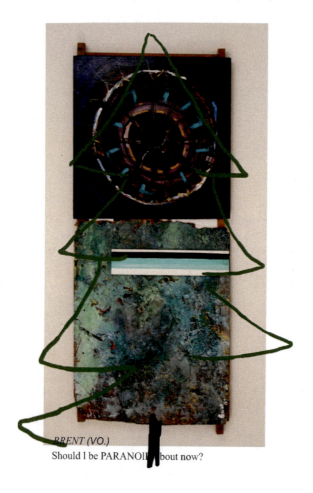

BRENT (V.O.)
Should I be PARANOID about now?

PETER (VO.)
Only if you WANT to be!

BRENT (VO.)
You are correct. It was also near where I egged the house before I knew it was the wrong thing to do.

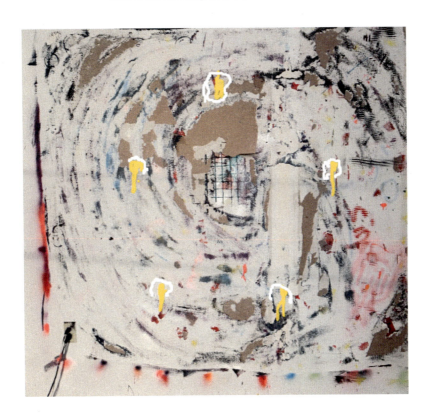

CHRIS (VO.)
Pete, did we have that fun tidbit?

[Pause]

Those eggs ruined the paint for many years after.

PETER (VO.)
That's a negative.

CHRIS (V.O.) (to Peter)
It is nice to know we don't know **it all.**

PETER (VO.)
So, we know you painted an image of a window in encaustic while at your childhood home.

BRENT (VO.)
Yep, in the driveway. I pulled out a portable camping stove and warmed up the wax right there NEXT TO THE PINE TREE! The wax was melted in my metal coffee maker from Europe.

CHRIS (V.O.)
Did you paint on canvas or wood?

BRENT (V.O.)
I think I recall it was on stretched canvas, maybe about 2.5' x 3.5'.

PETER (VO.)
So why paint the window?

BRENT (VO.)
It may have been one of the first times I knew good from bad. Or at least felt shame for breaking something.

CHRIS (V.O.)
Now we are getting somewhere. It's okay. What do you recall? Take as much time as you need.

BRENT (VO.)
There was a small yard and small parking lot. They were for our house and the duplex next door. The two-door garage was painted white, and was separate from both our house and the duplex. Anyway, Dad had asked what I wanted for my birthday. **1** wanted a slingshot.

CHRIS (V.O.)
Brent, do you remember how old you were?

BRENT (VO.)
Not exactly... 5, 6, 7?

CHRIS (VO.)
So you got a slingshot for your birthday?

BRENT (VO.)
It came in a white box with some kind of note from the maker.

CHRIS (VO.)
Pete, did you ever have a sl ings hot growing up?

PETER? (VO.)
Don't remember about a slingshot. But I had a BASEBALL BAT. Why, did YOU?

CHRIS (VO.) *(laughing)*
Brent, what do you remember about the slingshot?

BRE NT (V O.)
It was awesome. It was made of wood by a real, Cherokee, Native American. It had a red snake with black dots, on the handle.

PETER (VO.)
We have an idea where this is going, but it may be good for you to reflect on it.

BRENT (VO.)
I guess you know I broke the garage window?

CHRIS (VO.)
Suppose so, but that is okay. What were you aiming at?

BRENT (V O.)
I had aimed at the garage once, and the rock ricocheted off its concrete wall. On another occasion, I aimed at the large wooden door. I soon realized the force of the impact, and refrained from aiming at the garage. Dad told me that if I broke anything of value with the slingshot, I would get a spanking.

CHRIS (VO.)
Do you remember anything about the rock?

BRENT (VO.)
Gray and heavy, but not that big. God, it may have been a piece of GRANITE, but I don't know. My Grampa gave me some Granite that did come from Stone Mountain.

CHRIS (V O.)
What do you remember about the window itself?

BRENT (VO.)
Well, the garage was not used for the cars. It was a mess in there, and I ha rdly eve r go t to go i n.

CHRIS (V O.)
Okay, but what about the window itself?

BRENT (VO.)
It was almost completely black behind there. Mysterious, but kind of scary. Behind the win dow, was my dad 's s tuff.

CHRI S (V O .)
Hmmm ? How was the windo w actually broken?

BRENT (V O.)
I s tarted to pretend the rocks were airplane s and spaceships.

PETER (V O.)
Oh, boy.

CHRI S (V.O.)
That is the kind of thi ngs many boys do.

BRENT (V.O.)
I aimed the rocks into the air like I was launching them. I think I wanted to launch them over the garage, but that's speculative.

CHRIS (V O.)
On e went through the window?

BRENT (VO.)
With a big cras h. I was frightened. I instantly knew I had broken something important.

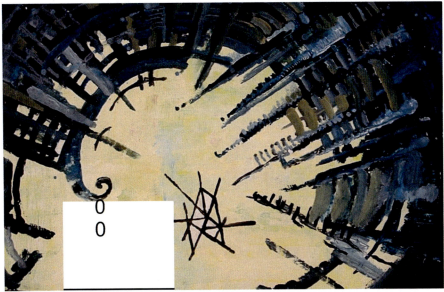

CHRTS (VO.)
You okay?

BRENT (V.O.)
Yeah, I am doing well, but the 02 in this cell room is not enough for the amount of people in here. There is no moving air. *(pause)* So, you KNOW what happened next!

CHRIS (VO.)
You got spanked.

BRENT (VO.)
Yes, but not right away. When I knew I had broken the window,
I went to see Mom immediately. I asked her if I was going to get a spanking.

CHRIS (VO.)
What did she say?

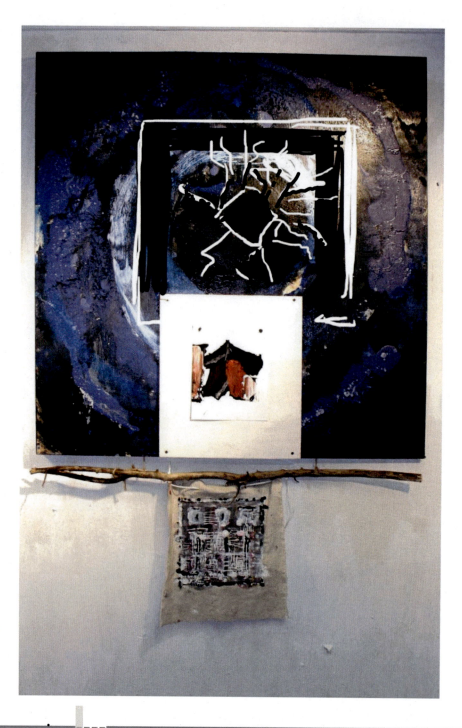

BRENT (VO.)
I really don't remember that conversation well, but something about the fact that, "We will have to wait and see when Dad gets home from work," and some comment about how I probably would.

CHRIS (V.O.)
A little time to think about it, ehh?

BRENT (VO.)
T felt horrible, and J hid.

CHRIS (V.O.)
Were you scared of your dad?

BRENT
He can be a serious man.

BRENT (V.O.)
OOPS! There are people in here.

CHRIS (V.O.
Don't worry about them; they probably won't remember you. Where did you hide, if you don't mind me asking?

BRENT (VO.)
No problem. But don't you know all this already? I hid under my sister's bed for hours. Dad came home, and they had to eat dinner without me.

CHRIS (V.O.)
They did look for you.

BRENT (V.O.)
Actually, I heard them yelling for me, looking for me. I felt even worse for hiding when I could tell they were getting really worried. Mom was in tears. It was a small house. Awhile after dinner, Mom knelt down next my sister's bed and found me. She was so happy to see me.

CHRTS (V O.)
And your dad?

BRENT (V O.)
I'm getting there. I don't remember that conversation very well either, but it went something like, "Son, we love you, but you really scared us tonight. First of all, you did break the garage window with the slingshot. Remember our deal? In essence you deserve a spanking for that, but that is not what concerns me most. The window is replaceable. What really bothered me was that you did not come when we called for you later. Did you hear us calling you? You frightened your mother pretty bad. In essence, you deserve a spanking for the window and for scaring us, but I am only going to give you one."

CHRIS (V O.)
Did he beat you?

BRENT (V.O.)
Hurt a little physically, but I would not say he beat me. I was spanked on the butt; I think with a Bolo paddle without the ball.

CHRIS (V O.)
A Bolo paddle? Is that a kind of toy?

BRENT (V O.)
Yep. I learned not to buy them 'cause when the ball broke off the rubber tether, it got confiscated and put on the shelf as the paddle.

CHRTS (V O.)
How did you feel after the spanking?

BRENT (VO.)
Dad tried a little preaching to me afterwards, but I felt totally abandoned.

CHRIS (V O.)
We know a little about your parents.

BRENT (V.O.)
Then you probably know that I only got a couple of paddlings at home while growing up. I don't even remember the other time, or times.

CHRIS (VO.)
Despite their faults, you have some great parents!

BRENT (VO.)
Yeah, when T did get a spanking in 8th grade at DeKalb Christian Academy, Dad came charging to my emotional rescue before the Headmaster. Dad did not like the reason I got spanked, or the fact that they were still doing it at that age. It may have been the last spanking at that school. Dad let them have it.

CHRIS (v.0.)
Forgiveness is a big thing when it comes to relationships. Brent, as you learn to forgive yourself and your family, just know you have also been adopted by a new family that may need forgiving at times, too.

BRENT(VO.)
Are you calling yourself part of my family?

PETER (VO.)
Not as much as YOU being a part of OUR family.

BRENT (V. 0.)
Excuse me, but T don't know if I would call your "group" a family; the Mob is also a family.

[Pause]

CHRIS (VO.)
Sure it is! But some families are healthier than others, and all have issues. And by the way, do you remember the etymology of yom name?

BRENT (VO.)
What has that to do with anything?

CHRIS (V.O.)
It's what your parents named you. It may mean nothing to you, but think about it.

BRENT (V.O.)
"BRENT" is an arctic goose, but in original English it means, "From the STEEP HILL."

[Pause]

BRENT (V.O.)
Oh, my gosh.

CHRIS (V.O.)
And "WESTON?"

BRENT (V.O.)
...WESTON means "of/ from the West."

CHRIS (V.O.)
"From the steep HILL in the West." I like that.

GUARD
BRENT WESTON.

BRENT
I'm over here.

GUARD
Come with me. We need to get your clothes changed for discharge.

Brent is the first one taken out of the room. He asks to go to the restroom. Guard points to a sink in a low lit, dirty, yellowish brown closet, down the hall. Brent is amazed the guard is trusting him to go down the hall by himself. He takes a pee in the sink next to the mops. He returns and thanks the sheriff. He is taken to another set of cells.
Guard calls many others out. Brent gets excited when the last one is called. If they follow the same earlier order, his name will be called next. He is given a bag with his stuff, and changes back into his shorts and tank top. His Bible is still in the backpack, but his sandals and Swiss Army Knife are gone. Someone hands him a small slip of paper with one Bible verse from *John*. It is typed in red.

                BRENT
You would not know what happened to my sandals?

                LA DY BEHIND COUNTER
You say you had some sandals?

                BRENT
YES!

Woman goes back behind a wall.

                LADY BEHTND COUNTER
Nope, sorry.

BRENT is ready to go, barefoot and all. But they start releasing people opposite the order taken from the last room. Brent knows now, that he still has to wait aw hile before they let him go. He has been told his paren ts are outside waiting, and he cannot wait to see them . But th e line of di sch arge is long and going slo w.

                BRENT (V O.)
Pe ter. You th ere?

                PETER (VO.)
Yes, sir.

                BRENT (VO.)
Will I get to talk to y'all anymore? The techn ology; I don't how,
or if i t wor ks, outside these walls.

                PETER (VO.)
Of course, but it may be more infrequent. You need to know your body and mind are not in a state that is acceptable to typical standard s of so ciety. It is going to be rough for you, but when

you need it the most, we will be there for you. Remember the circle with the dot.

Brent d raws a circle on the wall and punctuates the middle with a soft an d qui et, but solid, hit. He hears a tone in one ear and then the other.

                BRENT (VO.)
Chr is?

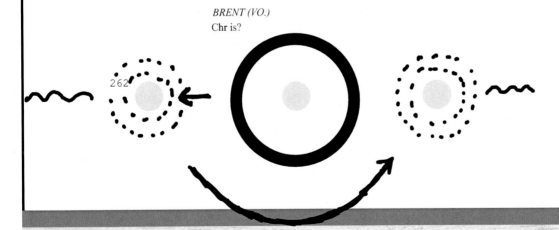

CHRIS (V.O.)
Believe me, I'll be there. I'm on YOUR case! I'm your number one connection. YOU are my main assignment, got it?

BRENT (V.O.)
God, I am literally the last one out of here. They have followed the exact order, but only reversed.

CHRIS (V.O.)
Man up, dude! The first will be last, and the last will be first.

Brent's name is immediately called. Brent is finally let out into the lobby with his backpack. He is barefoot. He is not seeing clearly, and thinks he hugs his parents. There is still paper work to be processed. He goes with his dad. His dad sits on a chair, and Brent climbs into his lap. For five minutes, he sits there in the lobby in his dad's arms quietly. Brent doesn't concern himself with what others think. He looks at his ring finger. The string is still there. It brings him back to the physicality of the world, and thoughts of £.

II. Leaving Confinement to Rest in Dad's Lap

EXT. LEAVING JAIL ----------- DAY

Eventually, the family walks out of the glass doors and past the Courthouse window that Brent had busted. Brent looks up at the sun, directly feeling its warmth. His eyes are extremely sensitive; they are blinking fast and squinting. His mind seems to have lost a tether. Brent feels the hot pavement on his feet; it reminds him of his other senses, and he smiles. Each stone on the gravel parking lot begins to hurt with each step.

BRENT
May I get a hamburger?

PARENTS
Sure, if that's what you want.

Brent senses something wrong with the lights inside the architecture of the fast food joint.

BRENT
May we take the hamburgers and go somewhere else to eat?

The family eats next to the water near the base of Stone Mountain.

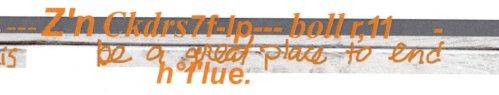

This be a great place to end h'flue.

INT BRENT'S PARENTS' HOUSE----- DAY

Brent walks through the door from the garage. He is barely glad to be home. He is extremely tired. Brent doesn't talk much, and eventually asks if he can lie down. His parents are very accommodating. Brent goes back to a real bed for the first time in weeks. His mind is skipping in thoughts. Linearity in normal thinking is gone. He can't sleep; he cannot stay awake.
Every 15 minutes, he is up and out of the bed. It is a vicious cycle. He goes to the piano
bench where he first saw E sitting. He sits down and presses a few keys. He finds three or four notes that ring true to him, and repeats them over and over, trying to add in other piano notes. He has no idea how to play the piano; he never had any lessons. He goes back to bed. Through the night, he just turns in bed. The graph-line images return to his mind like a slide projector that turns off and on in the most random patterns.

> CHRIS (V.O.)
> Rough night?

BRENT (VO.)
Urrrg. Get away. Y'all don't exist. But the images in my mind are too precise for y'all not to exist.

CHRIS (V O.)
I'll take that as an affirmative!

Brent's mind seems scrambled.

BRENT (VO.)
You come and go at your pleasure. When I want to communicate with you, I get nothing.

CHRIS (V O.)
It's important, RIGHT NOW, you now do something that you enjoy.

BRENT (V.O.)
I don't even know if you are real.

CHRIS (V O.)
You have not had a Coca-Cola in awhile!

BRENT smiles to himself, and goes to get one from the kitchen. There are no Cokes in the refrigerator, but several cans in the cupboard. He takes one, but does not open it.

CHRIS (V O.)
How about some music?

Brent goes back to his room and pulls out a small boombox and headphones.

CHRIS (V O.)
No headphones. We want you to take the boombox and put it on the counter in the bathroom and take a bath. And take the Coca-Cola with you.

BRENT (VO.)
ABATTTH?

CHRIS (V O.)
Yes, its been too long since you've just kicked back, listened to some music, and enjoyed some private space.

Jq. Hat Tub
Coc.q-C.014t ,n the

Hot Coca-Cola in Tub

INT. BATHROOM -----PARENTS' HOUSE -------------EVENING

Brent is drawing water for the tu b, and turn s on a pop radio station, B98 .5.

>BRENT (v. O.)
>Really not suppose to have a plug-in radio in the bathroom while taking a bath.

>CHRIS (V O.)
>Guess that puts your life in your own hands for the time being. You will be fine.

>CHRIS (V O.)
>How you feel ing, Brent?

>BRENT (V O.)
>Can't sleep ! How YOU doing?

>CHRIS (VO.)
>Ordered out CHINESE.

>BRE NT (V.O .)
>Chinese secret? Hmmm. Chinese FOOD sounds pretty good to me, about now.

>CHRIS (V O .)
>Enjoy your bath.

>BRE NT (V O.)
>Ts P eter a round?

>CHRTS (V O.)
>No, but T can call him up.

>BRENT (VO.)
>Up, from where?

>CHRIS (V O.)
>I could CALL him . He is not sitting at the COMM. If you want to talk to him, I can make it happen.

Brent is about to open his can of Coca-Cola.

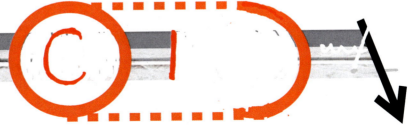

266

> CHRTS (V.O.)
> Have you ever had a HOT coke?

> BRENT (VO.)
> Not sure what you mean.

> CHRIS (VO.)
> Don't open the can! Drop it into the tub, under the spout.

> BRENT (VO.)
> That's pretty gross.

> CHRIS (VO.)
> Having it temperature hot, or because it's in a tub?

> BRENT (VO.)
> TUB!!

> CHRIS (V.O.)
> Leave it under the hot water until it gets noticeably hot. THEN, wash the can under the spout above the water level.

> BRENT (VO.)
> Ohhh?

Brent plays with an unopened Coca-Cola can in the tub for awhile until it is hot. Then he washes it, and has his first hot Coca-Cola while chilling to the radio.

> CHRIS (V.O.)
> When you have had about half a can of Coke, on the rim of the tub where you keep the shampoo and soap, I want you to do something. Turn the can at about a 45 degree angle, and balance it on the bottom rim of the can. Slowly take your hands off, but keep them close lest the can roll off into the tub. Trust me.

Brent does it, first try.

> BRENT
> Your signals must be coming through the radio.

No response and it is quiet for awhile, except for the pop songs. Brent's mind scrambles again. He gets out of the tub and puts some clothes on with no linearity of thought.

20. Baseball at the Private Mental Hospital

INT. LIVING ROOM PARENTS' HOUSE   **EVENING**

He walks out and finds his mom in the living room. She knows something is wrong.

>MOM
>Brent, you okay? Would you like to talk about it?

Brent nods his head for "yes."

>MOM
>Can you describe to me what's wrong?

>BRENT
>I can't sleep.

>MOM
>We noticed you seem a little anxious. Can you describe to me your thoughts?

>BRENT
>They are skipping. It's like a slide projector in my mind, and I cannot turn it off. *(Pause)* I think I'm being contacted through radio waves.

>MOM
>We love you, so it's okay to talk about these things. Would you say you're having thoughts that race uncontrollably?

Brent nods again. He puts his head slowly on his mother's shoulders.

>MOM
>You are going to be okay!

>BRENT
>Mother, please help. *(Pause)* Help me, please. My thoughts, they are too fast.

> MOM
>> Wednesday, we have set an appointment for you to see a doctor at a special hospital. It deals with these situations. *(Pause)* I made a birthday cake for you.

> BRENT
>> What day is it?

She hides that she is about to tear up, and smiles a little.

> MOM
>> It is Monday. We thought we would celebrate your birthday tomorrow.

Brent doesn't register. His eyes are glossy and close to tears.

> MOM
>> You think you can make it until Wednesday?

Brent silently shakes his head for "no," while his head is still on her shoulders.

> MOM
>> Do you think you need to go now?

Brent silently sniffles, and shakes his head for "yes."

> MOM *(Confidently)*
>> Okay. We will all get our things and go.

INT. BRAUNER HOSPITAL: ELECTROENCEPHALOGRAPH ROOM --------------- EVENING

> DIAGNOSTIC LADY
>> You must be Brent?

There is small chat as DIAGNOSTIC LADY is putting electrodes onto Brent's scalp. Brent lies down on the table and is freezing cold, reminding him of jail. Lady connects wires.

> DIAGNOSTIC LADY
>> That's unusual. Why is that string around your finger?

               BRENT
          It's a long, convoluted, love story. The string, l found in jail.

               DIAGNOSTIC LADY
          Fascinating. I want you to relax and try not to move.

               BRENT
          Okay.

               CHRIS (V O.)
          Hey Brent, I have Peter here with me. Tf you feel currents that are
          bothersome, dance with them in your mind. Remember the stillness
          when you were on the floor in jail and making art with the sound.

INT. WHITE JAIL (CLOSE UP: BRENT ON FLOOR) ----- NIGHT -------------FLASHBACK

[Flashback to the floor of jail.] Brent is drawing symbols very slowly on the floor.
Lifting a finger seems to change every current in his body. Brent feels as if he can play a
spider's web like a musical instrument, with the acupuncture like pressure points on the floor.

INT. BRAUNER HOSPITAL: ELECTROENCEPHALOGRAPH ROOM --------------EVENING

               CHRIS (V O.)
          You can use the table itself to release the tension. And remember,
          position of the hand. You can make a circle with the
          thumb and birdie finger on each hand, and interlock them during the
          test.

Machine is turned on. It does not hurt. However, someone shuts a door in the building, and
Brent's body shakes violently. Soon, the test is over. Diagnostic lady looks very
puzzled. She is looking over the machine with hidden concern.

               DIAGNOSTIC LADY
          Brent, something is not making sense with the reading.

               BRENT
          Is something wrong with the machine?

> DTAGNOSTTC LADY
> Sorry Brent, but l think l am going to need to run the test again.

> BRENT
> I'm very cold. May I have a blanket over me during the test?

Brent interlocks his birdie fingers and thumbs. Then he touches his big toes together. The test is soon over.

> DIAG NO STIC LADY *(Not wanting to alarm Brent with the results)*
> This o ne is better.

She takes off all the electro d es exce pt for two that are symm etrically oppo site each other.

> DIA GNO ST IC LADY
> Where did you say you got that strin g?

> BRENT
> DeKalb County Jai l.

The conversa tion goes fuzzy as Brent exits the room.

> BRENT (V O .) *(to Chris and Peter)*
> She left two electrodes on my head on purpose. She left them where frontal horns would be, or antennas on a robot from *Meet The Jetsons.*

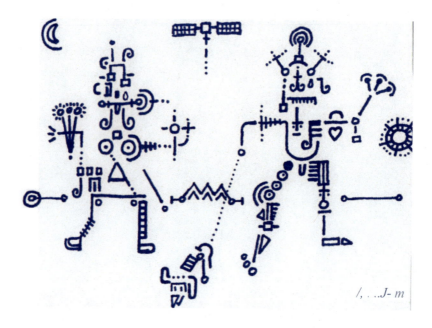

/, . ..J- m

PETER (VO.)
Don't worry about it.

CHRIS (VO.)
Just take them off when you get back to your room and throw them away.

INT. BRENT'S ROOM at BRAUNER --------NIGHT

Brent's room looks like a nice hotel room with two, single beds. It has its own temperature controlled air-conditioner. He has no roommate, and there are not many people on the unit. On the table next to him, he has brought a book by C.S. Lewis, *The Problem of Pain*. He is told to get some rest, but he is unable to get any continuity of sleep. He keeps adjusting the thermostat. A tall doctor dressed in a nice, gray suit with yellow socks and tie, and classy, black, leather shoes, comes in by himself. He is very kind. Brent's mom and dad are already in the room.

BRAUNER DOC.
Hi, Brent. I'm Dr. *(Joe Smith)*. How you doing?

BRENT (staring a little glossy)
I'm not sure.

BRAUNER DOC.
You are an artist?

BRENT
Yeah, I was painting a colorful series of established Atlanta restaurants, diners, and bars. The old guard working tables, and the multitudes of regular patrons, were on life's stage. Then it all suddenly happened. Everything was connected. It was as if I was living in a play.

BRAUNER DOC.
"Living in a play?" Hmmm? What kind of paint do you use?

BRENT
Gouache, an opaque water-color.

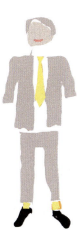

> DOC.
> Hmmm. Haven't heard of that one. It was not oil? I see in your records you are allergic to oil base paints. Is there anything else you think you could be allergic to?

Brent nods "No."

> BRAUNER DOC.
> It is my jo b to get you better. Do you know why you are here?

> BRENT
> My mind is not workin g right.

Doctor asks many more questions, but Brent is confused and overwhelmed with telling his story. Dad pipes in, and there is a brief conversation about where the doctor attends church. After awhile, the doctor and parent s leav e the room. The doctor comes back alone.

> BRA UN ER DOC.
> I have a couple of pills here that may help you get some rest. Would you be willing to take them?

> BRENT
> Have other people taken these pills before? Or am I a guinea pig?

> BRA UN ER DOC.
> These are newer d rugs, but we need to get the Alpha and Be ta waves at the right levels and under control.

> BRENT
> I don 't understand . Is that what she measured on that machine?

> BRA UN ER DOC.
> Yes. Would you like to see the results?

> BRENT
> Yes.

Doctor leaves and soon return s with a manila folder . Inside, is a series of se ismic like graphs. He shows the gra phs to Brent. He does not understand them. Brent doubt s they are eve n his results, but tries to read the red handwriting and marks.

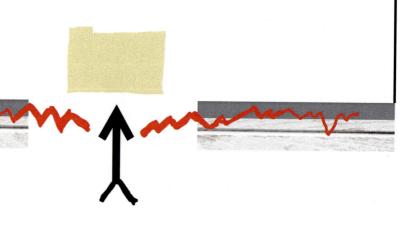

> BRAUNER DOC.
> Your natural brainwaves are not where they should be.

Doctor points to the lines and shows **him** the deficits and elevations.

> BRENT (Brent remembers Diagnostic Lady's name)
> (Jane Doe) seemed puzzled with the results.

> BRAUNER DOC.
> Who?

Doctor stares at Brent, a little surprised.

> BRENT
> The lady who read my brain waves.

> BRAUNER DOC.
> Oh, believe or not, I don't know the names of everyone who works here. I will let you know, there is a reading on here that I have not seen before. But let ME worry about that! For now, I would like you take these medicines and keep an IV in you for a little while.

> BRENT
> You know, when I was in jail, I was hypersensitive to sound, and thought I could hear some kind of radio frequency.

Brent asks if that technology is possible. There is a brief conversation about the CTA's tests earlier in the century.

> BRAUNER DOC.
> It is really crucial that you get some rest tonight.

Brent takes the pills and is soon asleep for a continuously *long* time. This is the first time in weeks. Brent awakens the next day on his own, and the nurses take out the IV. He is also given some more pills, along with a nice lunch.

INT. BRENT'S BRAUNER ROOM ---------**EVENING**

Brent is lying comfortably in his bed. He is chilling to faint sounds of a remote, Atlanta Braves baseball broadcast. His favorite announcers, Skip Carrey and Pete *van* Wieren, are callin g the balls and strik es in be tw ee n Coca-Cola commercials. About the 5th inning, the doctor arrives in his church suit and tie, with red socks. Mom also enters. The doctor starts asking questions.

      BRAUNER DOC.
      So Brent, how did you :;Jeep last night?

      BRENT
      I don't remember.

      BRAUNER DOC.
      How do you feel now?

      BRENT
      A little better.

      BRAUNER DOC.
      Ho w about this afternoon?

      BRENT
      I feel a little groggy, but okay.

      BRAUNER DOC.
      What did you do today?

      BRENT
      For the last hour and a half?

      BRA UN ER DOC.
      That will wo rk.

      BRENT
      I've been fading in and out of sleep, listening to baseball. It's good to hear Skip and Pete again.

The doctor looks perplexed, and his eyes dart to the right without really looking at anythin g. Deep breath from his morn. Brent knows something has gone wrong.

      BRAUNER DOC.
      From which direction do you hear the ga me?

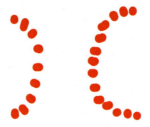

BRENT
I don't precisely know. I thought it was coming from the hall, but I'm not sure. It could have been coming through the wall, you know, from the next room over. It seemed to move around a little as to the source. It even sounded, at one point, like it was coming from above.

BRAUNER DOC.
Brent, this is a single story building. It did not come from above, and there is nobody in the rooms around you.

BRE NT
How close is the closest radio or TV?

BRAUN ER DOC.
There are no radios, and the TV room is way down the hall. I do NOT think you can hear the TV from here, but I will go down and check and see what they are watching. Why don't y'all rest for a minute.

Brent picks up *The Problem of Pain* by Lewis while the doctor is gone. The game goes quiet. The doctor soon returns.

BRAUNER DOC.
Brent, what you reading?

BRENT
The Problem of Pain by C.S. Lew is .

BRAUNER DOC.
What's it about?

Brent looks at the string on his finger and starts to tear.

BRENT
I'm not so sure, but I think good and evil, and personal pain, in context of losing his wife to cancer. I have not rea d it though.

BRAUNER DOC.
I think you should put the book down and not worry about that now. Why don't you wait awhile to read it.

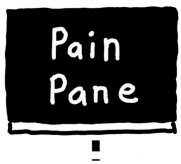

BRENT
How long?

BRAUNER DOC.
At least until you are fully better.

BRENT
How long is that going to take?

BRAUNER DOC.
I really don't know. Maybe not that long, but why don't you put the book down for a couple years.

BRENT
Seriously?

BRAUNER DOC. *(very politely)*
Yes, Brent. I went and checked. They have NOT been watching baseball in the lobby. We need to talk about what may be going on with you.

Brent nods.

BRAUNER DOC.
GMHT originally thought you were on a psychedelic, but changed their minds. I, too, am going to rule psychedelics out for now.
There are two illnesses that could be at play here; they may be inter related. One is called Bipolar, and one is Schizoaffective Disorder. The good news is that there are some effective
medicines to deal with both of these. They kind of act like a cast does to a broken bone, but just a cast for your neurotransmitters. The medicines help your mind link together properly. Combine the medicine and therapy, and I think you will be just fine. I
heard you were planning to hike part of the Appalachian Trail with a friend? Jim?

Brent nods again.

BRAUNER DOC.
I would like to get you to the point where you can do that.

Brent turns to Mom.

> **BRENT**
> Mom, have you heard of Bipolar and Schizoa-aahh what?

> **MOM**
> Yes. Schizoaffective Disorder and Bipolar ARE treatable. Glad we now have an idea this is it. There has been a lot of research in these fields. Bipolar is not necessarily a new thing for the doctors. Schizoaffective is just a word for a condition they better understand.

> **BRENT**
> I feel relieved that there are names for what I am going through.

> **BRAUNER DOC.**
> If you have any questions how the meds work, or any other question, feel free to ask. Also, we would like to keep you here awhile. Rumor has it you have a great insurance policy!
> Honestly, let us take advantage of it and make sure we get you as well as possible. Many people don't have the resources to really get this under control. You ARE fortunate.

> **BRENT**
> Maybe I can ask my questions tomorrow; I'm getting tired.

Brent looks at Mom.

> **BRAUNER DOC**
> That will be fine. But I'd like to start you on Lithium and Zyprexia as soon as possible.

Groggy, Brent looks at the doctor and really doesn't care.

> **BRENT**
> Okay.

Mom hugs Brent while he is still in bed.

> **MOM**
> Dad can come tomorrow. We will both be here during visiting hours.

Doctor and a concerned Mom soo n depart , wi th Mom asking man y questio ns.

Later, left in silence, Brent walks the long hallwa y double checking for a TV or radio.

He wants the final score to the Braves game. Arriving at a far-awa y TV room, people are trying to understand Kurt Cobain's suicide, while a few are engrossed in
Star Trek: the Next Generation 's, "The Nth Degree."

1. E ol\d *OrQ"9i"*•

EXT. REMOTE SUBURBAN COFFEE SHOP IN VIGINIA HIGHLANDS - 3 MONTHS LATER

E and Brent are sitting outside at a coffee shop by themselves. There is a roof overhead. Brent is so m ber. His beard has been shaven. We SEE them talking from a distance.
Brent seems to be looking beyond E, then looks at the string on his fing er. E is d rink ing red wine and Brent, an Oran gina.

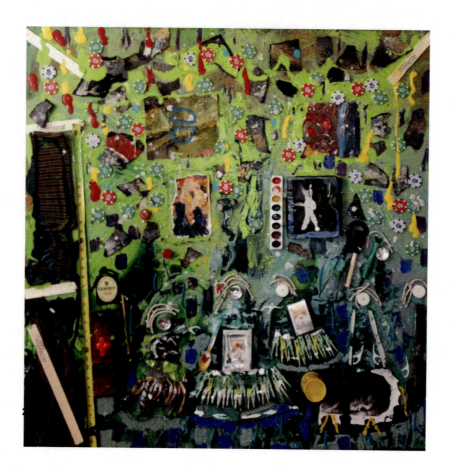

                    E.
            ... so why the string on the finger?

Brent pauses and looks directly at E, holding back tears.

                    BRENT
            It's a long story E, I honestly don't want to talk about that part very
            much.

                    E.
            That's okay Brent. We don't have to talk about anything you
            don't want to, and it's getting about time for me to go. Before I go,
            I want you to be one of the first to know that I am moving. I will
            soon be headed to San Fran... I think my art will be better received
            out there.

Brent looks down at the string.

                    BRENT
            £, I already knew that.

E. looks a little stunned.

                    BRENT
            E, do you remember those voices I briefly mentioned to you a
            minute ago, about when I was locked up? Whether or not they are
            real is another story, but they told me, emphatically, you were
            definitely moving to San Fran. In a sense, I have been emo
            tionally prepared for this moment dealing with you
            following YOUR dreams. I wish you the best.

They sit there quietly for a few minutes as the wind blows through the trees. A single dove noise is heard in the background.

                    E.
            I must go now.

They hug. The dove flies away.

INT. BRENT'S BEDROOM - NIGHT

Brent is in bed and takes the string off his finger. He looks out the dark window. The window turns bright. Birds are chirping.

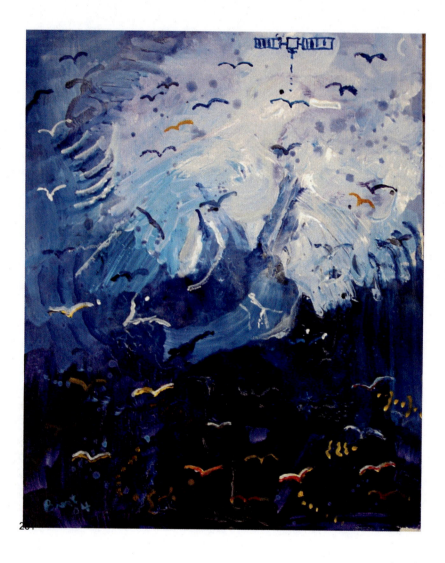

mi ?*aps*   s.\ill   c.on Jer:r
  +hrs   *hi:sv.*
  p:.tin4-t".j o.P *mine_*

My first
Acrylic in
Highschool

My "Pops" still considers
this his
fav. painting of mine.

→

5urpr1.se at Mailbox

12.

EXT. PARENT'S HOUSE MAILBOX

Brent opens a package from Jim. Inside is a pair of river, Jesus looking sandals. They are the exact kind that Brent had been wearing when arrested. There is a note. "Heard you 'lost' yours. I've had these since we worked the river together. Consider mine, YOURS now. Love Ya, J.!"

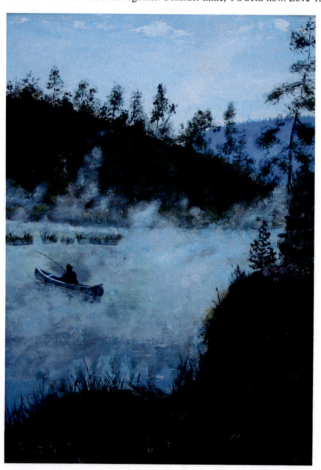

Finished: The story manically is now written in completion.

13. # C,vrrent' Artwork

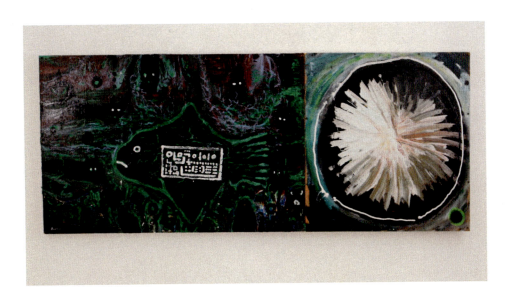

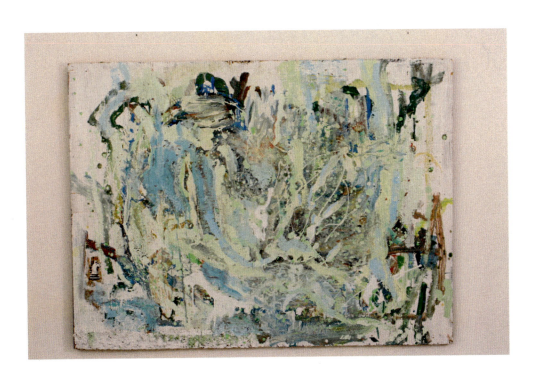

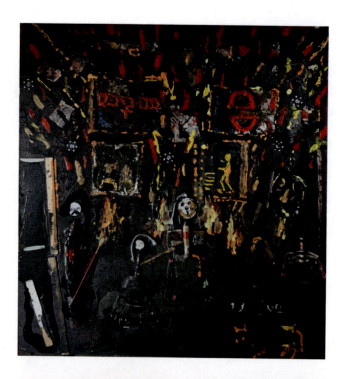

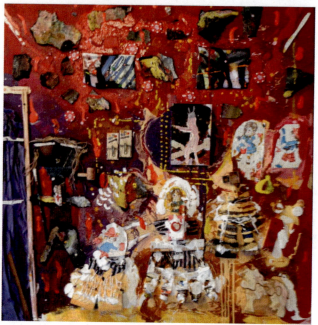

Las Meninas

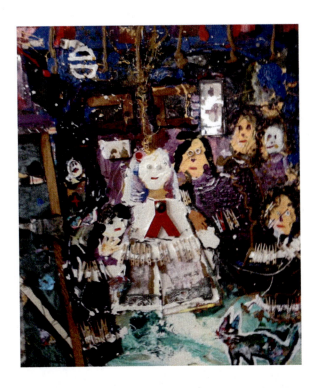

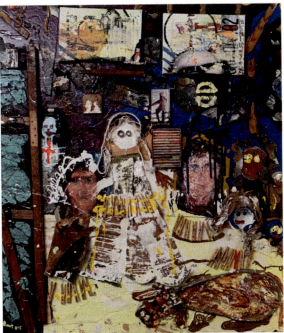

Las Meninas

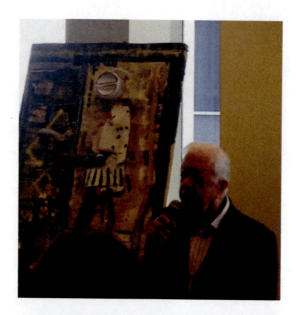
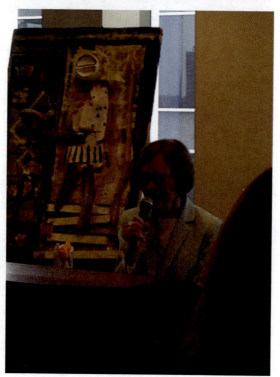

wti.Avf tr:> -ifles2 fo k.s-
fb,
th!4r **svpptrvr** •*n.* **cl2&J,·'j**
w(ᴀᴀ *,Ure,s.*

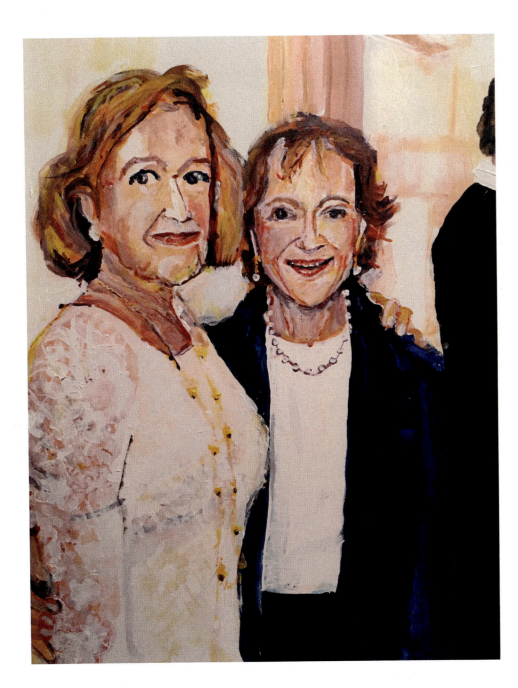

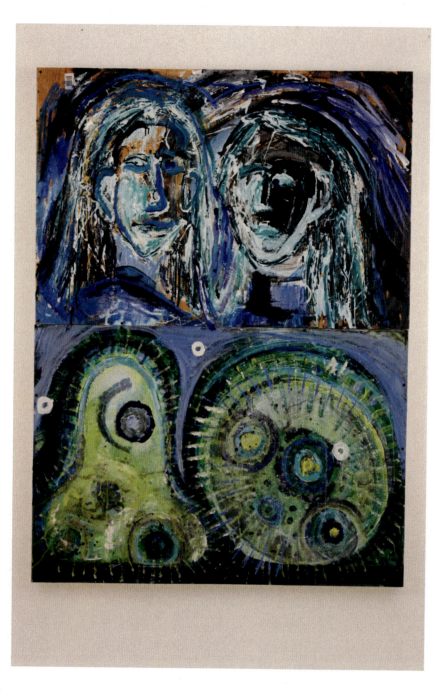

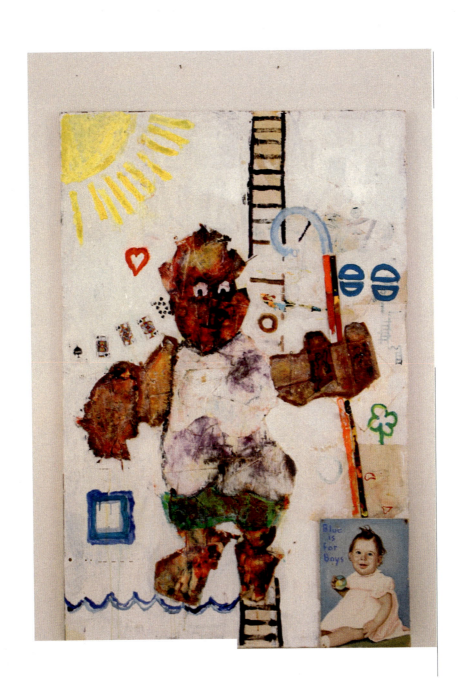

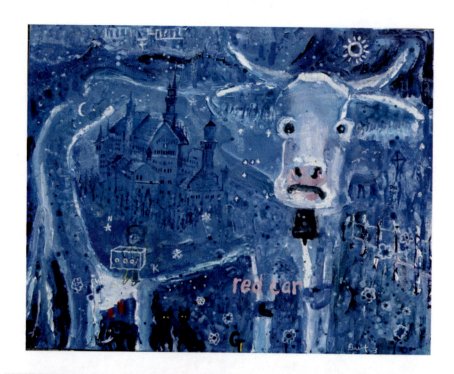
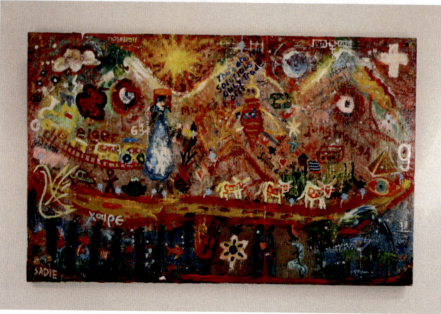

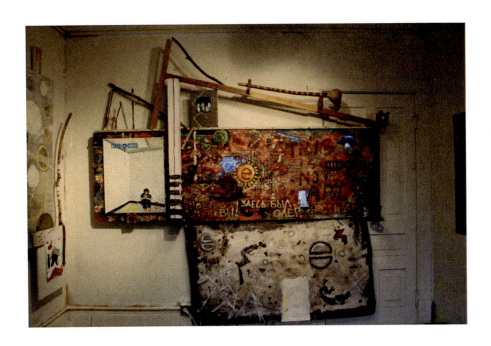

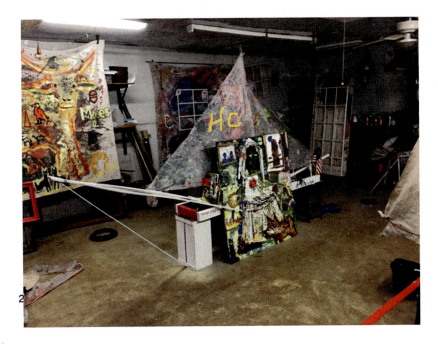

- self portrait table
- On a "Hill" of a wave

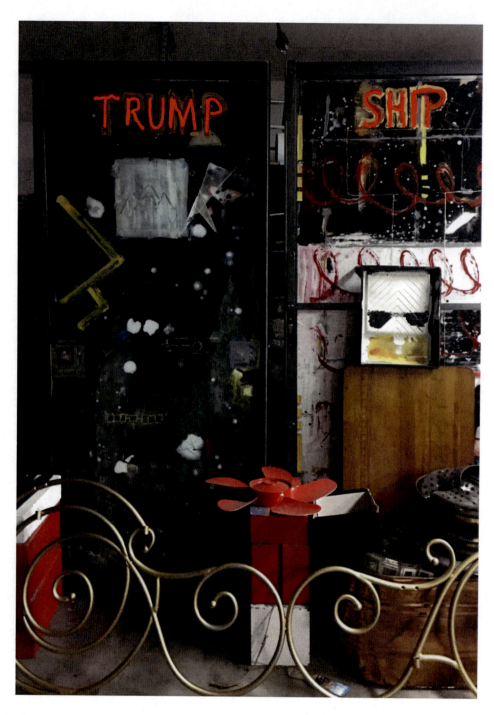

15. ff10.st   Rec.ent Works

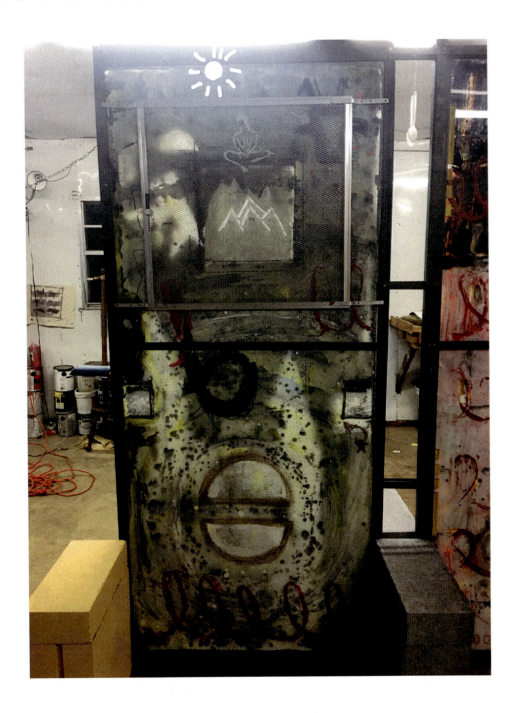

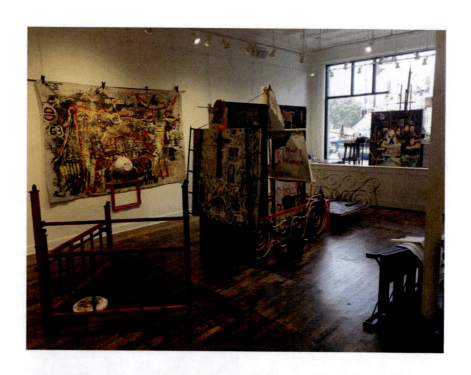

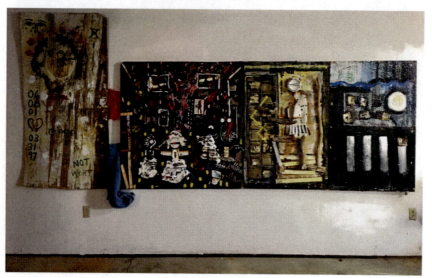

300

- Trump Ship
- Bernie kneels to the DNC

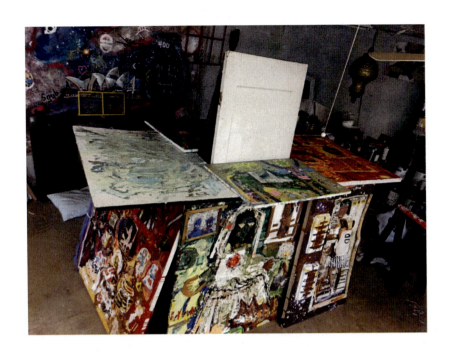

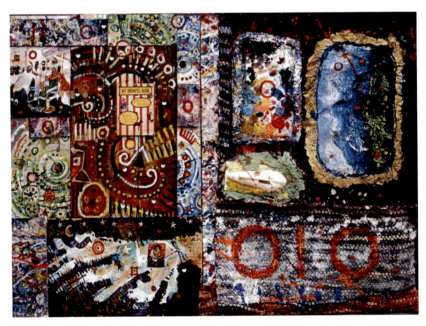

- House of Painted Cards
- The Tribe Speaks

+lutn , *is*... bd.e1e.

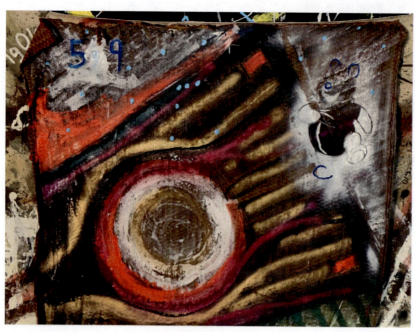

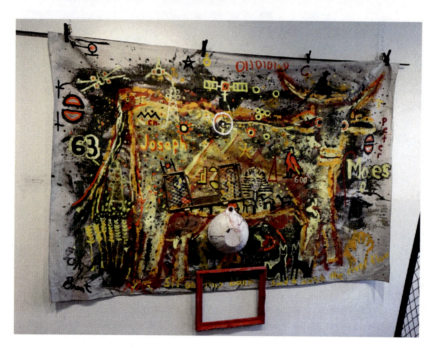

" *WA l,'ke* a *E'j,+1"',.)*eo:r v.{a*I k,..,w a&,.,-l*

Walk like an Egyptian, cause,"I know more about Isis than the Generals do! Believe me!"

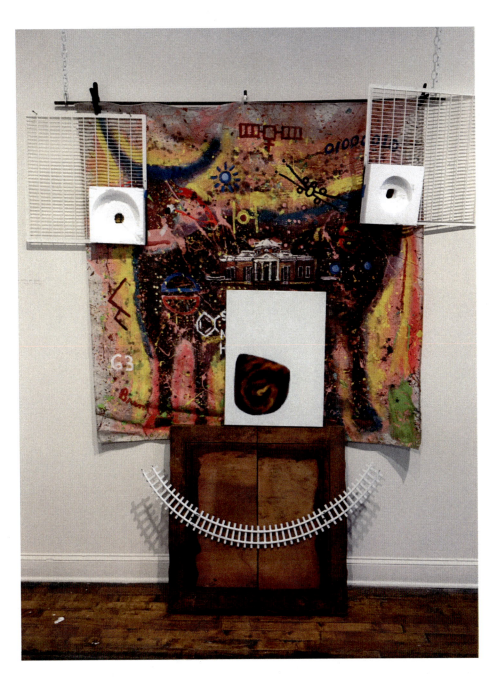

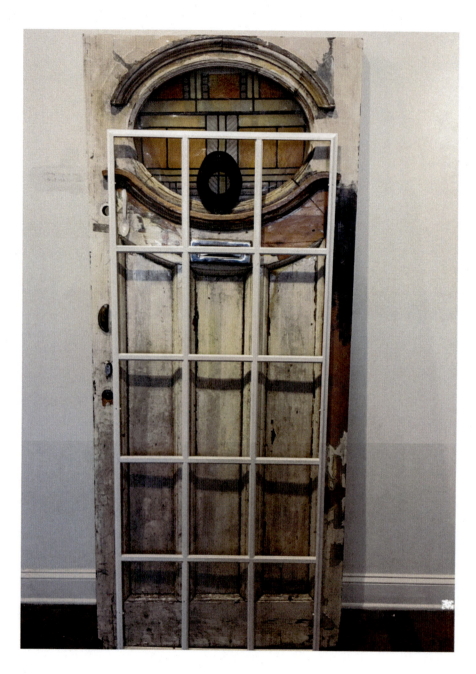

299

White House Window

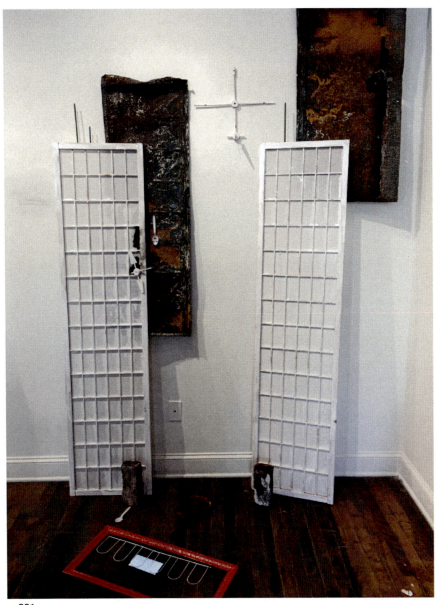

€.S u.S n6w we ove..-r:Ta
Jesr1s, how c:1<9   u..,e lo"e r,ur
Jesus how we love our enemies, r enemies.
Jesus, how do we love our enemies? eflenue.s-?

I'I. FinQl Notes

ft is obvious that through the years, I have rambled, tramped on, and wrestled wi th memories of an unorthodo x passage of incarceration. This has been an incredible spa rk and focus to create art. In simple language, I have always wanted to know what really hap pened to me so many years ago. Writing and paintin g has been a life force, and thera py to express my past and current dilemmas. The many years of depr essio n that followed jail time were eventuall y overcome, even with all my questions. Do I have an illness? Yes. Do I still communicate wi th Chris? On occasion I do. As rare as it is now, I even felt Peter talking to me the other night. Warning: this is crazy. I felt Peter specifically say there was a message to me that involved Pres. Obama, and Sara Bareilles. Go figure! It did not make since. I told my wife, I did not know much about Sara "B." I put Obama's and Sara B.'s names into Safari . I even told my wife in real time,"I am going to look this up." The second video that popped up was "Riveting Performance Sara Barflies Live singing 'You've Got a Friend' 2015 in HD." I had NEVER seen this video before! You ought to check out the visuals! My last name was in the photo behind Sara, while she sang on stage. On another front, do I still talk with E? On occasion. We are s till distant friends.

However, most important, I am learning what true love is abou t. I am not alone, and I am created for a good pur pose. Beneath my illness, beneath my manic fee li ngs toward *E,* and "above" Ch ris and Peter, are loves that run deep er. Genesis] :l g ives meaning to the universe. "In the beginning God created the Heaven's and Earth." The ma jes ty simply keeps the tears in my eyes and me humble. In my will and in my brokenness, I have chosen to taste and do good and evil in this world. I have been torn in two and have felt blessings and judgement. The knowledge that Christ is the bes t exa mple of Love, and the au thor of Love itself, is precious. Mercy gives hope!

God has used community,exercise, therapy, and medicine to lovingly bring me back into social "norm alcy." I ha ve been truly blessed with suppor tive family, Christian
communi ty along the way, lifelong friendships, and even Governme nt suppor t through a group started by Former First Lad y Rosalynn Carter. These people never gave up on me. Afte r the three week incarceration in 1994, I was finally able to graduate in 2012 from the University of Tennessee at Chattanooga. The social an d intellectual environment at UTC combined for an authentic, nurturing, and sustaining con tainer: to dialogue, paint, and perform. In 2012, I was asked to give a brief speech and introduce Mrs. Rosalynn Carter at a fundraiser in Atlant a. Mrs. Rosalynn Carter helped start an organization called *3Keys* that helped me find housing.

Lastly, in 2016, *I* got married to the love of my life, Je 1my. She has show n me mercy and lo ve beyond belief. She is my lo ver and friend i n o ne. I wa nt to thank Je nny for originally proof readin g this script. Her tremendou s support and love, despite my past, has brought more than a grin to my face. She has consoled, calmed, and brought passion to my heart and brain.

There are five recent paintings, dedicated to Jenn y. Two are cows she helped me paint. One is a painting I asked her to marry me with. The diamond ring was in a je welry bag hanging in the back of th e cradle. The forth paintin g is a "Unity Painting" we did live at our wedding to the song, *"All I Want is You"* by U2. The fifth was a Valentine's painting where we smeared pigments. It has a heart made of an upside down "j" and "b." The last images of thi s book are, "Isaac and Christ," a dove above my license plate, nails melted in a fire that destroyed over one hun dred uninsured paintings, a nut I found on my back step that a sq uirre l must have opened, a d rawing, my selfportrait, and my artist statemen t from the Senior Show before graduation

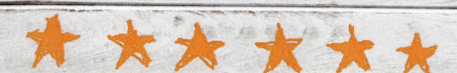

June 3, 2019

I will put in a journal entry for today. In other numbers it is 6-3-2019. I celebrate this day, in a weird way. In the past I have signed my art with the number 63. The 6 number is a lower case b and a "3" a sideways "w," my initials. My ringtone is ONE by my favorite band, U2. *Today* on my IPhone YouTube Channel came out a song by the band I just saw in concert, Snow Patrol. I really, really, enjoyed their concert. On the YouTube video, Snow Patrol came out and played live the song ONE with a cameo from Bono of U2 at Ward Park 3 Bangor, N. Ireland.

Giving credit to where it is due, I want to thank U2 for the two songs;

YAHWEH

"40"

The song"40" is one of my favorites now. Mike sang it at Jenny's and my wedding. God is in the process of restoring all that I lost, redeeming all the "locust has eaten."

Boston 2001 "Wowy and Bad and Wtshnn"

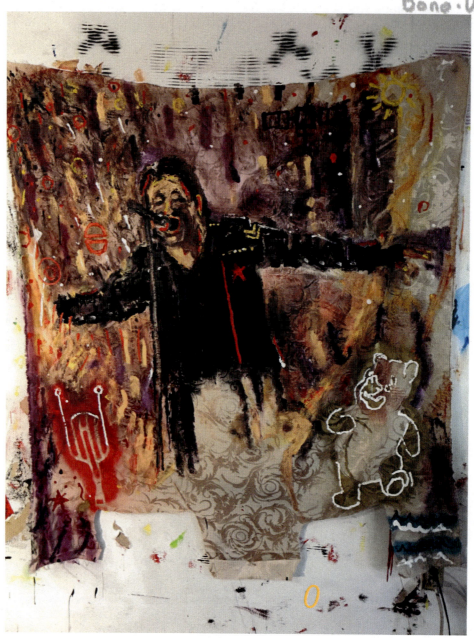

Bono·U2

Thank You Bon

The Edge - U2

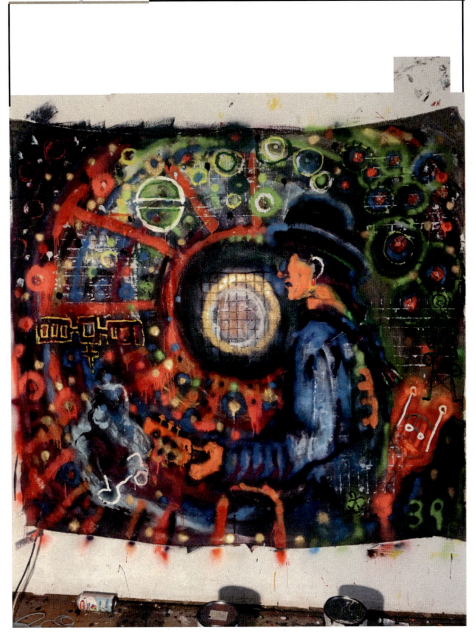

Thank You to The Edge

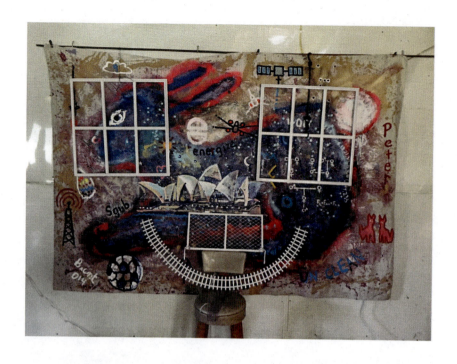

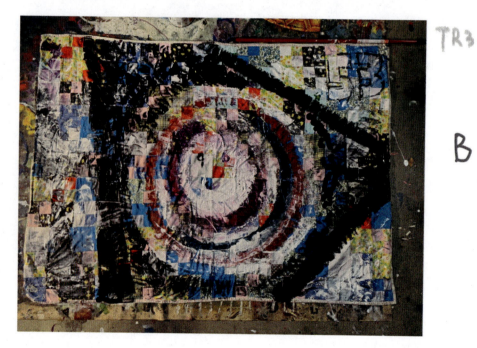

Black Balloon Makes Her Fly.

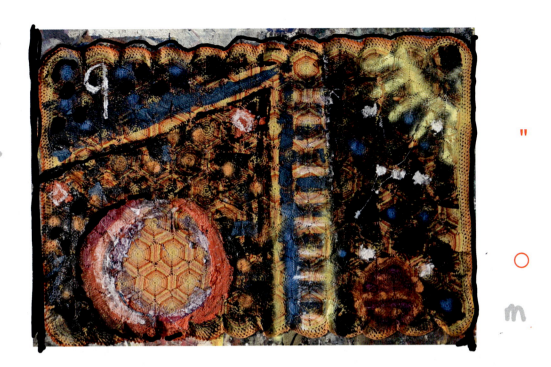

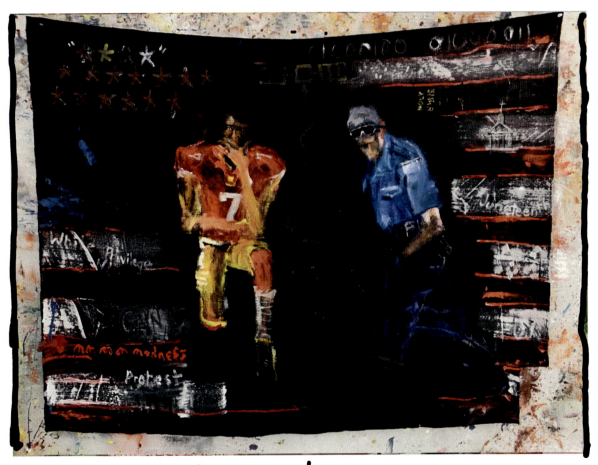

Need No Words

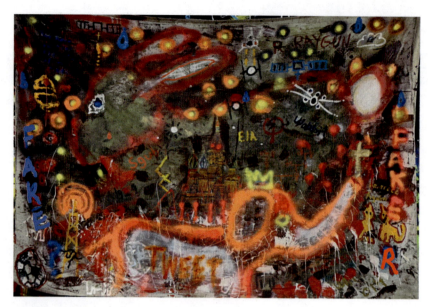

Patty cake, Patty Cake, Faker's Man   vrs

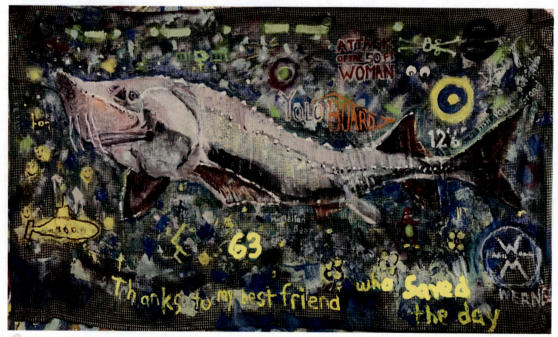

302   we all wish for a

Friendly Sturgeon

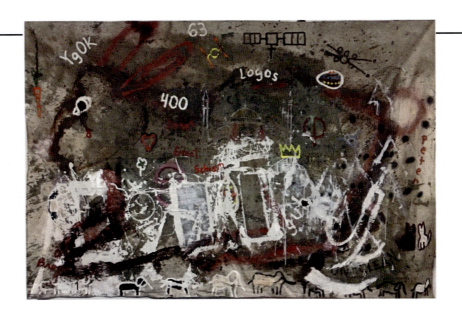

White Elephant Party

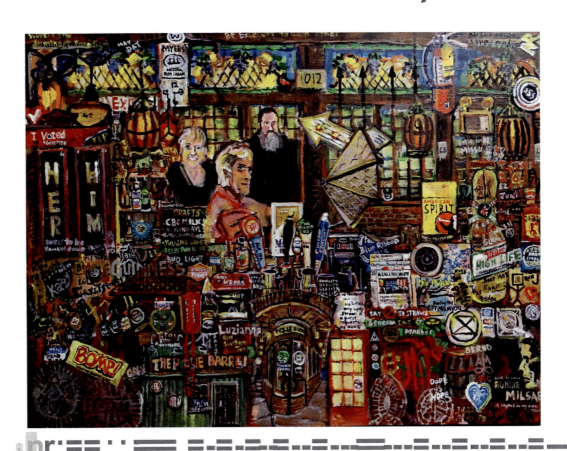

Dangling Carrot
"Bartender Please"

Zarzour's + Griffin's 2019

CHATTA

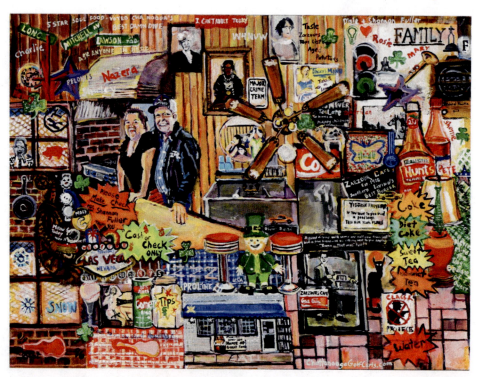

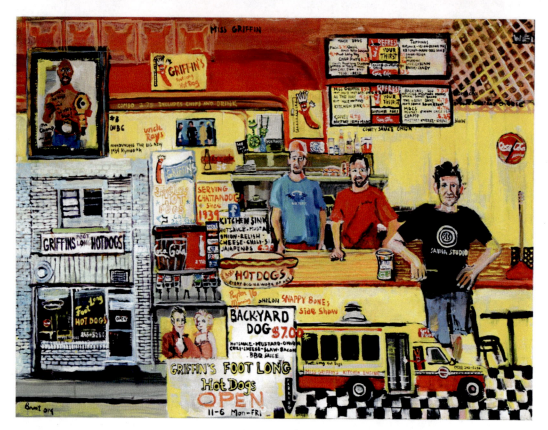

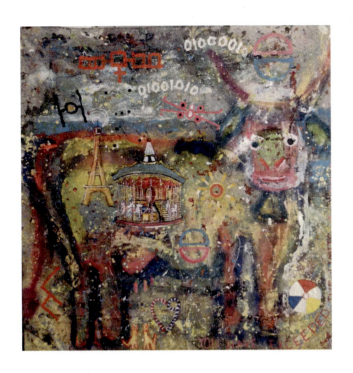
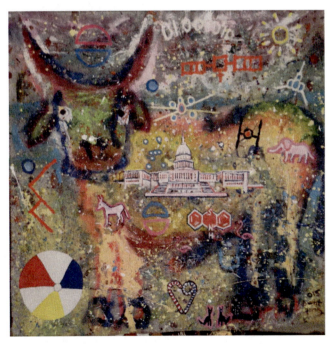

Jenny got a blister on her hand from throwing paint with brush

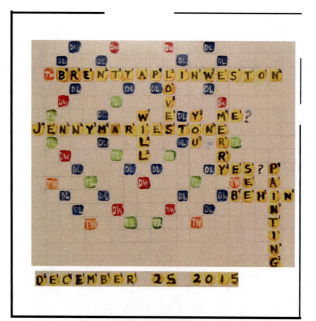

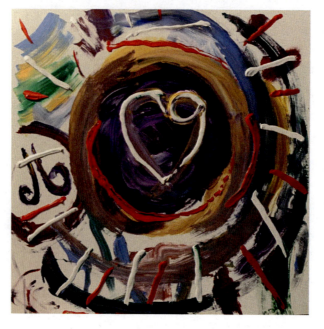

Engagement & Wedding Painting.
Painted to "All I want is You" (v.2) 6 minutes

11"e...

+f.e OG?ck *skpr:*

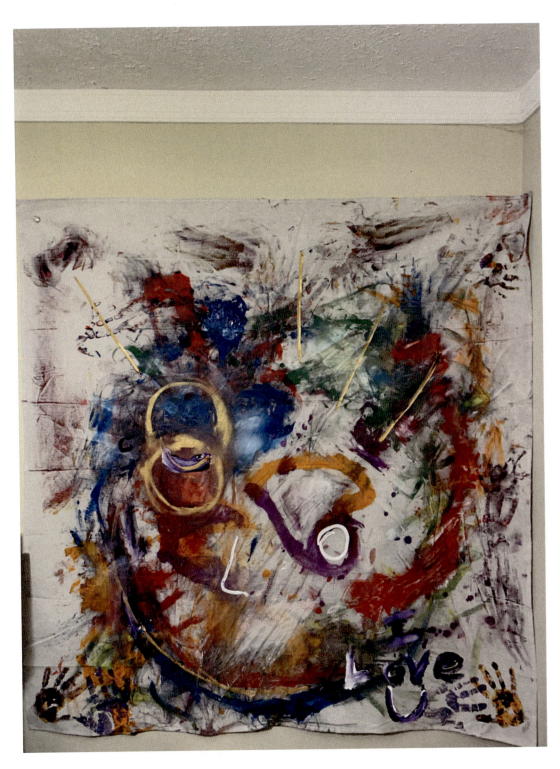

For Valentine's Day my wife wanted to do a painting together.

We had a great time making this art.

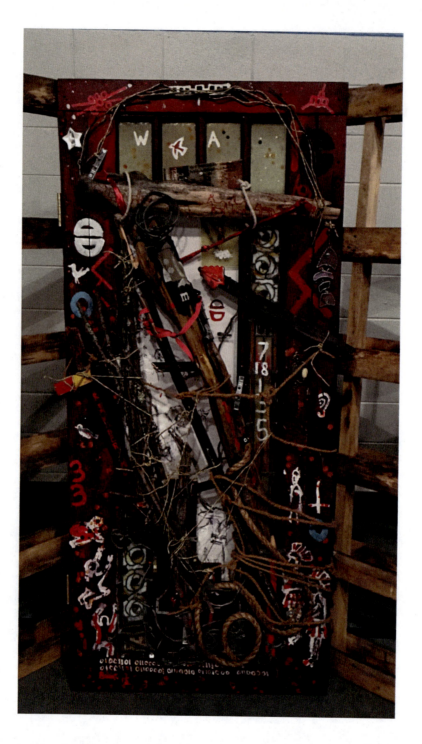

Isaac & Christ

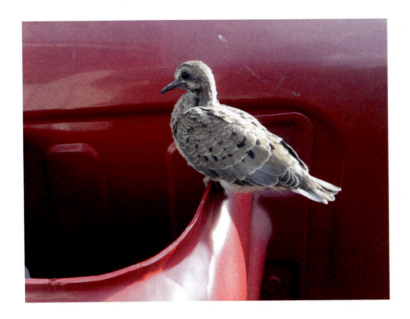
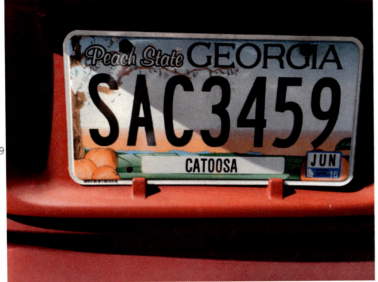

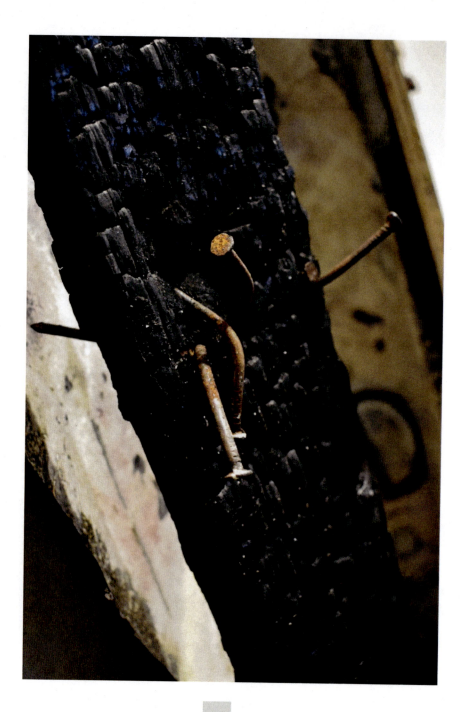

r::'rom t-f..e tire ct-f
ar ;,, s+rq_ge..
my

From the Thanksgiving Day warehouse fire that destroyed about 100 of my paintings.

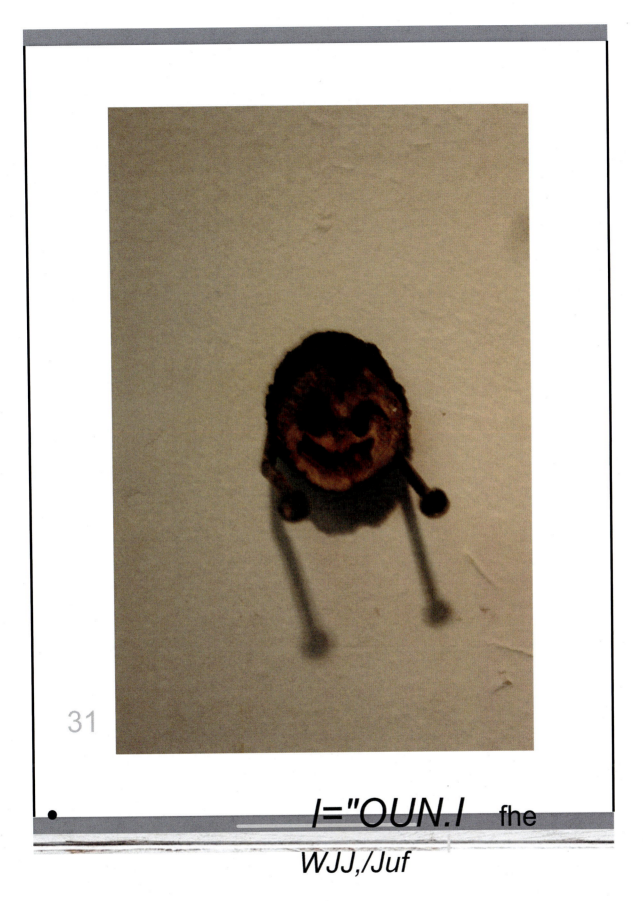

Wollie the wall nut. I found this on the back steps, and supported it on the wall by nails.

Op=-p[‘

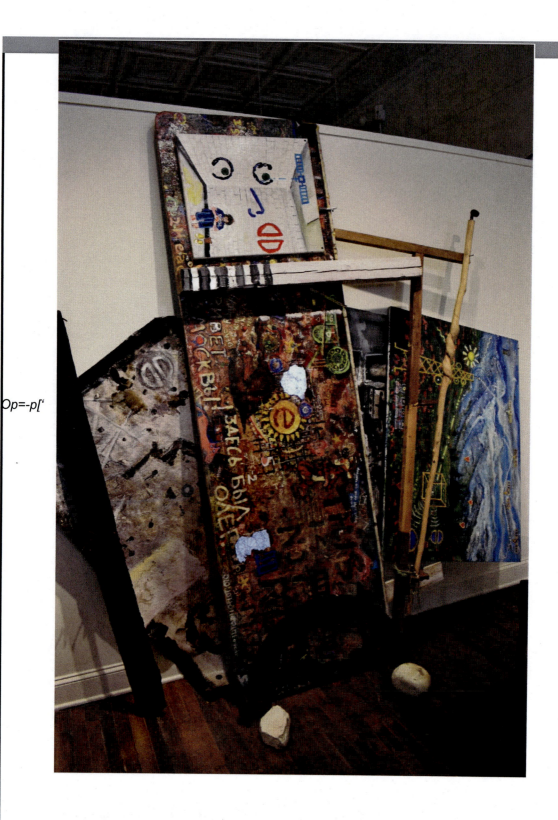

- self portrait table in recent show.
Muse Madness

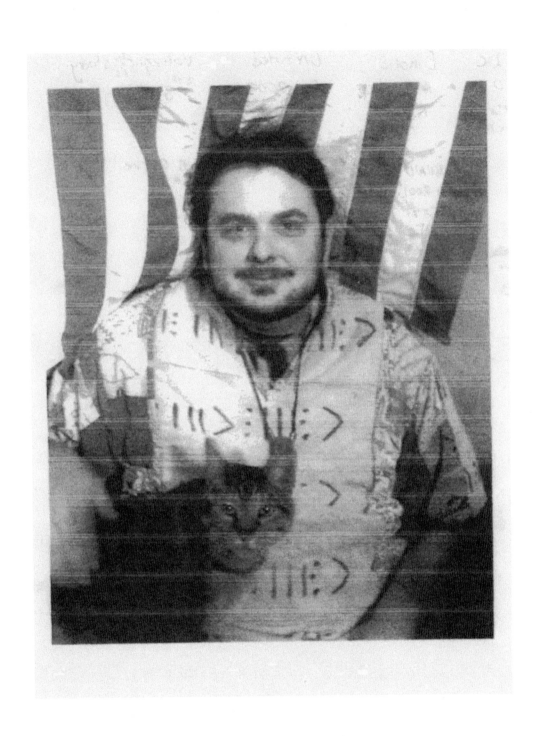

III II TJ-D-{(ill
---f

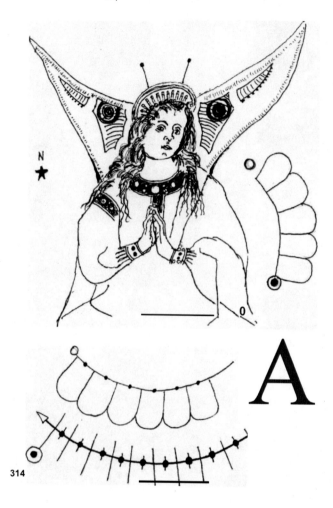

314

I for one.   Or is it two?

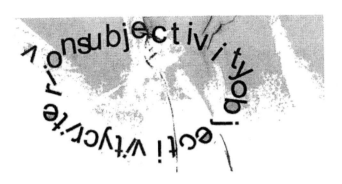

Yes I Think

Humpty Dumpty sat in his cells
Contemplating his broken shell,
All the Naturalist and Materialist men,
Tried to   put Humpty together again.

———————

But with his Creator held
And, the Creator's bond, "Arise
Humpty!"
"Walkon."

Made in the USA
Columbia, SC
27 May 2023